The ILIB
Lipid Handbook
for Clinical Practice

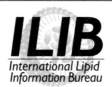

International Lipid Information Bureau

ADVISORY BOARD WRITING GROUP

Antonio M. Gotto, Jr., MD, DPhil
Chairman, ILIB Advisory Board
Dean and Provost of Medical Affairs
Weill Medical College of Cornell University
New York, New York

Gerd Assmann, MD
Professor of Medicine
Director, Institute for Clinical Chemistry
and Laboratory Medicine
Director, Institute of Arteriosclerosis
Research
University of Münster
Münster, Germany

Rafael Carmena, MD
Professor of Medicine
Department of Medicine
University of Valencia
Chief, Endocrine and Nutrition Service
University Hospital
Valencia, Spain

Jean Davignon, MD
Professor of Medicine
University of Montreal
Director, Hyperlipidemia and
Atherosclerosis Research Group
Clinical Research Institute of Montreal
Montreal, Quebec, Canada

Arturo Fernández-Cruz, MD
Professor of Medicine
Chief of Medicine
Director, Prevention and Rehabilitation
Center of the Cardiovascular Institute
Hospital Clinico
Complutense University
Madrid, Spain

**Jean-Charles Fruchart,
PharmD, PhD**
Director, Department of Atherosclerosis
Institut Pasteur de Lille
Lille, France

John J. P. Kastelein, MD, PhD
Co-Chairman, Department of Vascular
Medicine
Academic Medical Center
University of Amsterdam
The Netherlands

Rodolfo Paoletti, MD
Professor of Pharmacology
Dean of the Faculty of Pharmacy
Director, Institute of
Pharmacological Sciences
University of Milan
Milan, Italy

The ILIB is supported through educational grants from Parke-Davis, Division of Warner-Lambert Company, and from Pfizer, Inc. It is an educational effort intended to supplement governmental and other nonprofit efforts aimed at enhancing the dissemination of research findings and reducing the burden of cardiovascular disease throughout the world.

INTERNATIONAL LIPID INFORMATION BUREAU

The ILIB
Lipid Handbook
for Clinical Practice

Blood Lipids
and Coronary Heart Disease
Second Edition

Antonio M. Gotto, Jr., Gerd Assmann,
Rafael Carmena, Jean Davignon,
Arturo Fernández-Cruz, Jean-Charles Fruchart,
John J. P. Kastelein, and Rodolfo Paoletti

International Standard Book Number: 0-9646411-2-7

Additional copies of this handbook may be obtained from:

International Lipid Information Bureau
c/o Antonio M. Gotto, Jr., MD, DPhil, Chairman
Room F-105
1300 York Avenue
New York, NY 10021, USA
Telefax 1-212-746-8424

C ONTENTS

To the Reader	vii
Acknowledgments	viii
Abbreviations	ix

1 INTRODUCTION — **1**

2 CLINICAL GUIDE: Stepwise Approach to the Evaluation and Treatment of Dyslipidemia in Adults — **37**

2.1	Screen for dyslipidemia	40
2.2	Identify and characterize dyslipidemia	42
2.3	Perform full clinical evaluation	46
2.4	Estimate the level of overall CHD risk	48
2.5	Treat any underlying conditions and replace or reduce any drugs that can cause secondary dyslipidemia	52
2.6	Determine any primary dyslipidemia	54
2.7	Determine the need for dietary intervention and other lifestyle measures	58
2.8	Instruct the patient in the cholesterol-lowering diet and risk factor reduction	60
2.9	Consider and select lipid-regulating drug therapy as necessary	64
2.10	Monitor lipid-regulating interventions	69
Chart 2-1	Lipid Managment for Primary Prevention of CHD in Adults—ILIB Recommendations	70
Chart 2-2	Lipid Management for Secondary Prevention of CHD in Adults—ILIB Recommendations	71

3 CASE STUDIES — **73**

Table 3-1	Absolute Risk Estimates for ILIB Primary-Prevention Adult Cases According to PROCAM and Framingham Risk Calculators	103

C ONTENTS   (Continued)

APPENDIXES

A   **Sources: Major Adult Clinical Recommendations**   **106**

    A.1   Guidelines of the Second Adult Treatment Panel
of the U.S. National Cholesterol Education Program   106

    A.2   Recommendations of the Second Joint Task Force
of European and Other Societies on Coronary
Prevention   113

B   **Population Subsets**   **115**

    B.1   Management of Dyslipidemia in Adults with
Diabetes Mellitus   115
        Chart B.1-1 Evaluation and Treatment of
Lipid Disorders in Adults with Diabetes Mellitus—
ILIB Recommendations   134

    B.2   Management of Risk in Children and Adolescents   135

    B.3   Special Considerations in Women   147

    B.4   Special Considerations in the Elderly   156

C   **Characterizing Dyslipidemia**   **165**

    C.1   Determining Blood Lipid Values   165

    C.2   Common Causes and Presentations of Hyperlipidemia   168

    C.3   Obtaining Family History   170

D   **Elements of Lipid-Regulating Therapy**   **171**

    D.1   Lipid Effects of Lifestyle Changes   171

    D.2   Implementing a Heart-Healthy Diet   172

    D.3   Management of Overweight and Obesity   179

    D.4   Exercise Recommendations   183

    D.5   Smoking Cessation   189

    D.6   Lipid-Regulating Pharmacotherapy   191

    D.7   Other Treatment Options   203

    D.8   Tactics for Enhancing Compliance
with Lipid-Regulating Therapeutic Regimens   204

    D.9   Cost Effectiveness of Lipid-Regulating Therapy   205

E   **Pathophysiology**   **211**

    E.1   Summary of Lipid Metabolism   211

    E.2   Evolution and Stabilization of Atherosclerotic Lesions   220

F   **Additional Risk Issues**   **228**

    F.1   Risk for Stroke   228

G   **Additional Resources**   **231**

    G.1   Online Resources   231

Index   233

This handbook is intended for the general clinician in need of a straight-forward guide to the evaluation and treatment of blood lipid disorders in reduction of risk for atherosclerotic disease. The handbook synthesizes essential material from European and U.S. clinical guidelines and was for-mulated by an international group of experts, including lipid clinic and laboratory directors, after extensive discussions of issues and options in the management of dyslipidemia. As a consensus document, it represents the judgments arrived at by most of those concerned. The ILIB Writing Group hopes that the reader will find the handbook a simple and practical tool for understanding management recommendations in this field, and a way to share in the authors' clinical experience. It is hoped that with this handbook close to hand, physicians and other healthcare workers will not miss opportunities to intervene against cardiovascular risk factors.

The authors recognize that coronary heart disease prevalence and mortality trends vary widely around the world. Major improvements have evolved in some countries in parallel with marked deterioration in oth-ers, the epidemiology of coronary heart disease being greatly influenced by changes in national health policies, public awareness of risk factors, implementation of preventive measures, and medical education. As with any guidelines, the ILIB recommendations should be considered and applied in context, taking into account the resources available.

The handbook begins with a brief review of the status of low-density lipoprotein cholesterol, high-density lipoprotein cholesterol, and plasma triglyceride in the assessment of risk for coronary heart disease. A step-by-step guide then leads the clinician through the evaluation and treat-ment process, and is followed by 14 case reports that facilitate practical application of the treatment recommendations. To complete the hand-book, an appendix provides additional detail about action limits and treat-ment options and includes useful tips and reminders, as well as brief summaries of lipid metabolism and the pathogenesis of atherothrombo-sis. The Appendix also highlights the very important area of CHD risk prevention in subpopulations, including patients with diabetes mellitus, children and adolescents, women, and the elderly. A section new to this edition addresses the cost effectiveness of lipid-regulating therapy.

The Board's data review for the current edition ended November 7, 1999. Scientific findings published since that date are not included.

ACKNOWLEDGMENTS

The ILIB Writing Group wishes to thank the following individuals at Baylor College of Medicine for assistance in the preparation of the handbook: Suzanne Simpson, BA, who edited the handbook and assisted in its drafting, and Peter H. Jones, MD, Henry J. Pownall, PhD, Lynne W. Scott, MA, RD/LD, Christie M. Ballantyne, MD, Bassem el-Masri, MD, Joel D. Morrisett, PhD, and David P. Via, PhD, for helpful commentary. The help of Robert Dufour, MD, in reviewing the manuscripts at the Clinical Research Institute of Montreal is gratefully acknowledged, as is review by Alberico Catapano, PhD, of the Institute of Pharmacological Sciences in Milan, and Paul Cullen, MD, MSc, FRCPI, of the Institute for Clinical Chemistry and Laboratory Medicine in Münster. The creativity and dedication of Barbara Robin Slonevsky and her staff at Materia Medica/Creative Annex (New York), responsible for the design and production of the handbook, are deeply appreciated.

ABBREVIATIONS

ACE	=	angiotensin-converting enzyme
ADA	=	American Diabetes Association
apo	=	apolipoprotein
ATP II	=	second Adult Treatment Panel of the NCEP
b.i.d.	=	*bis in die* (twice a day)
BMI	=	body mass index
CABG	=	coronary artery bypass grafting
CHD	=	coronary heart disease
CVD	=	cardiovascular disease
DBP	=	diastolic blood pressure
EAS	=	European Atherosclerosis Society
ECG	=	electrocardiography or electrocardiogram
EDTA	=	ethylenediaminetetraacetic acid
ERT	=	estrogen-replacement therapy
FCH	=	familial combined hyperlipidemia
FH	=	familial hypercholesterolemia
GI	=	gastrointestinal
HC	=	hypercholesterolemia
HDL-C	=	high-density lipoprotein cholesterol
HMG-CoA	=	3-hydroxy-3-methylglutaryl coenzyme A
HTG	=	hypertriglyceridemia
IAS	=	International Atherosclerosis Society
IDL	=	intermediate-density lipoprotein
ILIB	=	International Lipid Information Bureau
LDL-C	=	low-density lipoprotein cholesterol
Lp[a]	=	lipoprotein[a]
LV	=	left ventricular
MI	=	myocardial infarction
NCEP	=	U.S. National Cholesterol Education Program
NS	=	not statistically significant
PTCA	=	percutaneous transluminal coronary angioplasty
PVD	=	peripheral vascular disease
SBP	=	systolic blood pressure
TC	=	total cholesterol
TG	=	triglyceride
TIA	=	transient ischemic attack
t.i.d.	=	*ter in die* (three times a day)
VLDL	=	very low density lipoprotein

INTRODUCTION

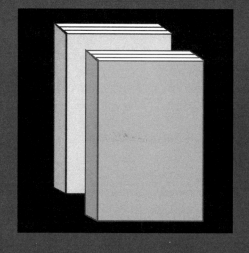

1 Introduction

1.1 Risk Overview

During recent decades, CHD mortality rates have fallen substantially in some industrialized countries, in particular Australia, Canada, New Zealand, the United States, and some European nations. The decreases are attributable to improvements in the presence of major risk factors and in medical care. In the cohort of the **Framingham Study** (United States), one third to one half of the 44% decrease in the CHD death rate observed in men between 1950 and 1989, and more than one half of the 51% decrease in women could be attributed to improvements in risk factors in the cohorts (Sytkowski et al. *Am J Epidemiol* 1996;143:338–350). Estimates for the U.S. situation nationwide are similar: reductions in risk factors could account for 50% of the marked drop in CHD death rate between 1980 and 1990, and improvements in other treatments could account for 43% of the decline. Seventy-one percent of the improvement was in patients with CHD and 25% could be explained by primary prevention (Hunink et al. *JAMA* 1997;277:535–542). For the population of The Netherlands, 44% of the 1978–1985 decline in CHD mortality rate could be attributed to primary prevention (Bots and Grobbee *J Cardiovasc Risk* 1996;3:271–276). In the **North Karelia Project** (Finland), a 48% reduction in age-adjusted CHD death rate among the middle-aged subjects was achieved through ensuring decreases across 20 years in plasma cholesterol (from a mean of 275 to 224 mg/dL, or 7.1 to 5.8 mmol/L), smoking (from a prevalence of 52% to 32%), and blood pressure (from a mean of 147/92 to 143/84 mm Hg) (Ginter *Bratisl Lek Listy* 1997;98:67–72).

Yet despite the elucidation of major risk factors, the availability of an effective armamentarium to control many of them, and the elaboration of cogent public health strategies and clinical management guidelines, CHD remains the leading cause of death in many developed nations, including the United States and most European nations. In many Central and Eastern European nations, prevalence is alarmingly high for hypercholesterolemia, hypertension, smoking, obesity, and alcohol abuse, and CHD death rates are increasing enormously. World Health Organization statistics (*The World Health Report 1998*) show that circulatory diseases, responsible each year for 5 of 12 million deaths in developed countries and for 10 of 40 million deaths in developing countries, are the largest threat to health for most adults. More than 7 million of the 15 million cardiovascular disease deaths worldwide are from CHD. Furthermore, the prevalence of CHD is increasing as populations age, and in some countries (e.g., in some Asian countries) as unhealthy lifestyles are adopted. Although many cardiovascular deaths are premature, an improvement in the quality of life of the elderly, with postponement of the onset of chronic illness to compress years of morbidity, is increasingly a priority.

In addition to the need for fuller compliance with population strategies to improve the healthfulness of diet and to ensure adequate physical activity and a tobacco-free environment, there are significant shortfalls in the implementation of clinical practice guidelines. Physician adherence, like patient compliance, is crucial for the effectiveness of preventive medicine. Even though lipid-lowering therapy is now considered an essential component of CHD prevention both in patients with and without established atherosclerotic disease (i.e., secondary and primary prevention), many physicians have not done an adequate job of ensuring that patients who could benefit from such therapy actually receive the treatment they require or receive adequately vigorous treatment.

According to estimates based on 1991–1994 data from the U.S. **National Health and Nutrition Examination Survey** (NHANES III), 65% of American adults eligible for cholesterol-lowering dietary or drug therapy are receiving no therapy of any kind. Only 1.4 million, or 6.6%, of 21.1 million drug-eligible U.S. adults are receiving such therapy (Hoerger et al. *Am J Cardiol* 1998;82:61–65). A number of surveys have described failure to reach NCEP cholesterol goals in patients receiving treatment. In Canada, the **Clinical Quality Improvement Network** investigators found that only 28% of 3,304 hospitalized patients at high risk for future cardiovascular events had lipid values recorded during their hospital stay or any time between 1988 and 1993. Cholesterol-lowering diet or drugs were prescribed for 22% and 8% of all patients, and women and the elderly (>70 years) were significantly less likely to have their lipids measured or to receive lipid-regulating therapy (Clinical Quality Improvement Network Investigators *Am J Cardiol* 1995;76:570–573).

The **EUROASPIRE** (European Action on Secondary Prevention through Intervention to Reduce Events) survey conducted in the Czech Republic, Finland, France, Germany, Hungary, Italy, The Netherlands,

Slovenia, and Spain found a high prevalence of modifiable risk factors in patients with a history of CHD (CABG, PTCA, acute MI, or acute coronary ischemia without infarction). Only 32% of the subjects were receiving lipid-lowering drugs, and among those, although patient compliance would also play a role, TC remained >213 mg/dL (>5.5 mmol/L) in 49% and >251 mg/dL (>6.5 mmol/L) in 13%. Among all the subjects, TC remained above those values in 44% and 14% (EUROASPIRE Study Group *Eur Heart J* 1997;18:1569–1582). The **Asian–Pacific CHD Risk Factor Collaborative Group** found that across 10 countries in the Asian–Pacific region, cholesterol was unmeasured in 1–58% of patients within 6 months of hospital admission for MI or unstable angina. Among the patients with TC ≥213 mg/dL (≥5.5 mmol/L), only 1–32% by country received formal dietary advice, and 6–60% received lipid-lowering medication (Keech *Atherosclerosis* 1998;136:S31 [abstract]).

Thus, despite fears of some critics of excess use of lipid-regulating drugs, it seems clear that there is underutilization by both providers and patients. There are significant gaps in control of other risk factors and the use of other categories of CHD prophylactic drugs as well. Physicians have the opportunity and responsibility to promote preventive measures such as smoking cessation and prevention, blood pressure control, weight control, regular physical activity, a healthy diet, management of the risk of diabetes mellitus, and, in secondary prevention, antiplatelet therapy. Even when the task of providing preventive services is delegated to other members of the healthcare team, the physician must set and support the agenda. These focuses are imperative in light of our improved therapies and substantially increased understanding of the pathophysiology of atherothrombotic disease. Preventive cardiology services need to be efficiently and comprehensively organized, and intensified efforts need to include those to increase patient compliance. (See Appendix D.8 for tactics to enhance compliance with lipid-regulating therapeutic regimens.)

1.2 Multiple Risk Factors

Although the focus of the ILIB is dyslipidemia, no CHD risk factor or category of risk factors should be judged in isolation. Control of multiple risk factors (see 2.4) is crucial in this multifactorial disease, and clinical practice guidelines now emphasize global risk. Risk factors tend to cluster and to interact synergistically. Among 350,564 U.S. men screened as possible participants in the **Multiple Risk Factor Intervention Trial** (MRFIT), only 3% were considered to be at low risk for CHD because of TC <182 mg/dL (<4.7 mmol/L), SBP/DBP <120/<80 mm Hg, and absence of current smoking, diabetes, or history of MI. Twelve years after screening, these men had an 89% lower CHD death rate, 53% lower total mortality rate, and an estimated increase in longevity of >9 years compared with the rest of the men (Stamler et al. *Cardiology* 1993;82:191–222). Similar differences in outcome according to risk factor levels were found in women in the **Chicago Heart Association Study** (*ibid.*). Data from follow-up through 1992 of U.S. men and women in **NHANES I** (1971–1975) (Figure 1.2-1) showed the presence of three major risk factors to triple the risk for a CHD event and nearly to double the risk for dying of any cause. Having four or five risk factors increased risk for a CHD event by five times and risk for death by three times during the 20 years of follow-up (Yusuf et al. *Prev Med* 1998;27:1–9). When any risk factor is present in a patient, it is important to assess for other risk components and to be vigorous in treatment of all of them.

Multivariate risk calculators that estimate 8- or 10-year absolute risk for a CHD event in adults without known CHD (primary prevention) include those developed from findings of the **Prospective Cardiovascular Münster** (PROCAM) study (also called the **Münster Heart Study**) and the **Framingham Study** data set. Both data sets represent long-term, prospective observational studies, chiefly in middle-aged, white subjects. The PROCAM risk algorithm is available in interactive format on line at www.chd-taskforce.com. Internet access to the most recent Framingham elaboration (Wilson et al. *Circulation* 1998;97: 1837–1847) is at www.nhlbi.nih.gov/about/framingham/riskabs.htm (or for a preliminary interactive site [accessed November 7, 1999] see www.usnews.com/usnews/nycu/health/sfheart.htm). Such tools mimic the multifactorial nature of CVD risk but do not replace full clinical evaluation. Not all major risk factors are included because of both theoretic and practical considerations, and it must be remembered that the presence of a risk factor may not confer high absolute risk over the next 8–10 years but will confer high risk during a lifetime of exposure. Individuals who are at high risk because of multiple marginal abnormalities in major risk factors

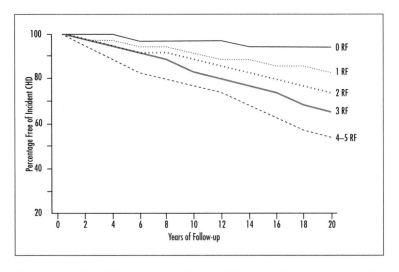

Figure 1.2-1. Probability of not developing CHD, according to number of risk factors, in follow-up (through 1992) of the first U.S. National Health and Nutrition Examination Survey (1971–1975). Risk factors considered were TC ≥240 mg/dL (≥6.2 mmol/L), current smoking, hypertension (SBP ≥140 mm Hg, DBP ≥90 mm Hg, or taking antihypertensive medication), diabetes (self-reported), and overweight (BMI ≥27.8 kg/m² for men, ≥27.3 kg/m² for women). Among the 12,932 subjects, 25%, 33%, 28%, 12%, and 2% had 0, 1, 2, 3, or 4–5 of these risk factors. From Yusuf HR, Giles WH, Croft JB, et al. Impact of multiple risk factor profiles on determining cardiovascular disease risk. *Prev Med* 1998;27:1–9; used with permission.

may be falsely reassured by estimations based on categorical risk factors. It is of great interest that the PROCAM risk algorithm for coronary events also identifies patients at high risk for stroke (see Figure F.1-1).

Major risk factors delineated for CHD have both strength of epidemiologic association and biologic plausibility. They should not be confused with risk associations based on preliminary or even trivial data, a distinction that is often ignored in media reports and that is misunderstood by many patients.

1.3 Dyslipidemia and Risk for CHD

Genetic, pathologic, laboratory, and observational and interventional epidemiologic studies have clearly established the primary role of plasma lipoproteins in the development of atherosclerotic CHD. Lipid risk factors encompassed by current clinical practice guidelines to reduce risk for CHD are LDL-C (and/or TC), HDL-C, and fasting TG concentrations. Lipid accumulation in the artery wall—from LDL, considered the key atherogenic lipoprotein, and perhaps from remnants of the TG-rich lipoproteins—is requisite to formation of the fatty streak (see Appendix E.2). A high concentration of HDL particles may to some extent counteract the lipid accumulation through enabling removal of artery wall lipid deposits. One hypothesis holds that the most important contribution of other risk factors, such as smoking and diabetes mellitus, is to promote plaque progression and rupture.

1.3.1 TC and LDL-C

The extensive observational epidemiologic data that relate elevation of TC or LDL-C to increased CHD incidence are from both between- and within-population studies. There is remarkable consistency among large cohort studies, and CHD risk has traditionally been considered to be 2–3% lower for each 1% decrement in TC concentration. However, Law et al. (*BMJ* 1994;308:367–373) on meta-analysis of international studies found a 10% difference in TC to be associated with about a 38% difference in CHD mortality rate. The international studies avoided regression dilution bias and were not influenced by the underestimation affecting cohort studies. At 25 years' follow-up of the classic **Seven Countries Study**, late CHD death rates remained largely accounted for by differences in serum cholesterol during the early phase of the study (Menotti et al. *Eur Heart J* 1997;18:566–571). In the **Ni–Hon–San Study**, the best-known migration study, middle-aged Japanese men living in Japan (Nippon), Honolulu, and San Francisco had progressively higher serum cholesterol and CHD death rates as lifestyle became progressively westernized, including a shift toward a diet higher in animal fat (Benfante *Hum Biol* 1992;64:791–805). At 27- to 42-year follow-up in the **Johns Hopkins Precursors Study**, TC concentration measured early in adulthood in men was strongly predictive of CVD in midlife. Risk for MI was increased five times in the highest compared with the lowest TC quartile, and a difference of 36 mg/dL (1.0 mmol/L) in initial TC concentration was significantly associated with increased risk for death before age 50 (Klag et al. *N Engl J Med* 1993;328:313–318). Such data are corroborated by experiments in animals in which pathologically typical atherosclerosis develops when plasma LDL-C concentrations are increased by high-fat diets. The genetic "model" of severe, premature atherosclerosis in humans is homozygous familial hypercholesterolemia, in which LDL-C concentrations exceed 600 mg/dL (16 mmol/L) and symptomatic CHD typically occurs by age 20 years.

In addition, as reviewed below, clinical trials using lipid-lowering drugs have unequivocally demonstrated that lowering LDL-C yields significant reductions in both morbidity and mortality from CHD in patients with or without established CHD, including in patients with only average cholesterol values for westernized societies. Moreover, LDL-C reduction as secondary prevention significantly increases survival, and it is likely that the benefit would occur with cholesterol reduction in general populations in modernized societies were trials feasible.

1.3.2 HDL-C

That HDL-C concentration is an independent and powerful inverse predictor of CHD incidence has been firmly established by numerous observational epidemiologic studies, which have indicated that risk for CHD decreases 2–3% for each 1 mg/dL (0.03 mmol/L) increase in HDL-C after correction for other CHD risk factors.

Information on the effects of increasing HDL-C in humans is limited but suggests favorable effects on CHD risk. Results of the 5-year **Veterans Affairs Cooperative Studies Program High-Density Lipoprotein**

Cholesterol Intervention Trial (HIT), the first completed clinical endpoint trial directly testing the hypothesis of increasing low HDL-C, included a significant 22% decrease in the primary endpoint of nonfatal MI or coronary death (p = 0.006), as well as decreases of 11% in death from any cause (NS), 25% in confirmed stroke (NS), and 59% in TIAs (p <0.001) (Rubins et al. *N Engl J Med* 1999;341:410–418). The beneficial effect of gemfibrozil therapy did not become apparent until about 2 years after randomization. Need for coronary revascularization was not significantly affected. Gemfibrozil therapy (1,200 mg/day) compared with placebo in HIT yielded significant changes in HDL-C (+6%) and fasting TG (-31%) but no significant change in LDL-C. Subjects were 2,531 men with CHD who had HDL-C ≤40 mg/dL (≤1.0 mmol/L), LDL-C ≤140 mg/dL (≤3.6 mmol/L), and TG ≤300 mg/dL (≤3.4 mmol/L). Optimum benefit with gemfibrozil was attained when on-treatment HDL-C was ≥35 mg/dL (≥0.9 mmol/L), even in the presence of high plasma TG (Robins et al. *Circulation* 1999;100[suppl I]:I-238 [abstract 1237]).

In the smaller, angiographically monitored **Lopid Coronary Angiography Trial** (LOCAT), also conducted in men with low HDL-C as the predominant lipid abnormality, gemfibrozil therapy retarded the progression of coronary lesions and the formation of bypass graft lesions (Frick et al. *Circulation* 1997;96:2137–2143). The favorable angiographic results achieved with the gemfibrozil therapy were similar to those achieved in trials using HMG-CoA reductase inhibitors (statins) in patients with higher LDL-C concentrations. (See also the BECAIT and BIP trials in "Plasma TG," next, regarding HDL-C raising.) Indirect support is available from some of the clinical trials testing LDL-C reduction, including the Helsinki Heart Study and LRC-CPPT (see below), in which treatment-induced increases in HDL-C were independently associated with a reduction in CHD events or decreased coronary lesion progression. Post hoc analysis of **Lipoprotein and Coronary Atherosclerosis Study** (LCAS) data showed patients with low HDL-C to receive the greatest angiographic and clinical benefit (Ballantyne et al. *Circulation* 1999;99:736–743). The coronary event benefits in AFCAPS/TexCAPS (see below) occurred in men and women who had reduced HDL-C as an enrollment criterion.

Low HDL-C often reflects HTG, obesity, a sedentary lifestyle, cigarette smoking, or impaired glucose tolerance. Low HDL-C may also be inherited, but not all individuals with inherit low HDL-C develop premature CHD (see Table 2.6-1).

1.3.3 Plasma TG

In the relation of fasting plasma TG concentration and CHD risk, some researchers have suggested that the conventional epidemiologic approach be abandoned in favor of a focus on metabolic and molecular mechanisms. In addition to the challenges posed by the marked intra-individual variation in fasting TG values, the various TG-rich lipoproteins have a close relation to the metabolism and composition of HDL and LDL particles and are considered heterogeneous in atherogenic potential. Measurement of subfractions or assessment of postprandial dynamics rather than fasting TG values may be needed in risk assessment. Moreover, the TG-rich lipoproteins are closely linked to blood coagulation and fibrinolysis. Since the 1980s, a variety of mechanisms whereby TG-rich lipoproteins may be atherogenic and prothrombotic have been identified.

In many earlier prospective studies, the predictive value of fasting TG tended to diminish or even disappear when HDL-C, coagulation factors, or indicators of abnormal glucose metabolism were considered. A number of analyses published in the past few years, however, have supported independent risk factor status. In 8-year follow-up of the prospective **Copenhagen Male Study**, relative risk on multivariate analysis for a first CHD event was increased 50% for the middle third of fasting TG concentrations and more than doubled for the highest third of concentrations, and a clear gradient of risk according to TG value was seen within each HDL-C tertile (Jeppesen et al. *Circulation* 1998;97:1029–1036). Analysis of 8-year data from the **Münster Heart Study** (PROCAM) showed the significant correlation between fasting TG and major coronary events (Figure 1.3-1) to remain after adjustment for LDL-C and HDL-C, even after other risk factors were taken into account (Assmann et al. *Am J Cardiol* 1996;77:1179–1184). Meta-analysis of 17 prospective population-based studies showed an increase of 88.5 mg/dL (1.0 mmol/L) in fasting TG to be associated with 32% and 76% increased risks for incident

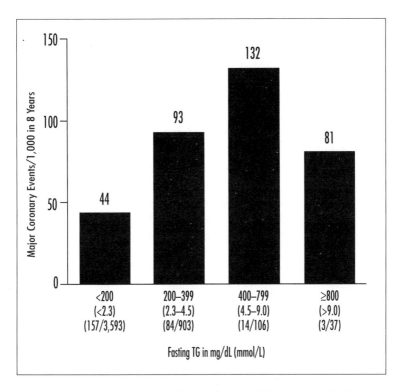

Figure 1.3-1. Incidence of major CHD events per 1,000 men (aged 40–65 years) in the Münster Heart Study (PROCAM) over 8 years according to fasting TG concentration. There were 258 events among 4,639 men. Very high plasma TG concentrations are associated with the presence of chylomicrons. From Assmann G, Schulte H, von Eckardstein A. Hypertriglyceridemia and elevated lipoprotein[a] are risk factors for major coronary events in middle-aged men. *Am J Cardiol* 1996;77:1179–1184; used with permission from Excerpta Medica, Inc.

CHD in men and women (Hokanson and Austin *J Cardiovasc Risk* 1996;3:213–219). Adjustment for HDL-C and other risk factors attenuated the risks (to 14% and 37%) but did not render them nonsignificant. HDL-C and fasting TG are both more important risk predictors in diabetes mellitus, and there is evidence that HDL-C, fasting TG, and diabetes each are more important risk factors in women than in men.

It is clear that not all forms of HTG impart the same risk for CHD. For example, HTG accompanying familial combined hyperlipidemia, type III hyperlipidemia, diabetes mellitus, central obesity, or a family history of CHD appears to be linked to the development of premature CHD. Some of the genetic disorders, however, that give rise to HTG (e.g., lipoprotein lipase deficiency and apo C-II deficiency, which lead to chylomicronemia) are not typically associated with increased rates of CHD. Although chylomicronemia has only rarely been linked to increased CHD risk, treatment of very high TG is needed to reduce risk for pancreatitis. Fasting plasma TG elevation in the approximate range of 150 to 250 mg/dL (1.7–2.8 mmol/L), and even up to 500 mg/dL (5.6 mmol/L), is frequently indicative of the cardiovascular metabolic syndrome (see below).

Indirect evidence for benefit of TG reduction is available from some lipid-lowering trials, including the Helsinki Heart Study and the Stockholm Ischemic Heart Disease Secondary Prevention Study (see below). It is possible that in these trials unmonitored LDL particle size was favorably affected as well. In LDL-lowering trials monitored by angiography or B-mode ultrasound, specific TG-rich lipoproteins (e.g., IDL) and markers of their metabolism (e.g., apo C-III) were key correlates of atherosclerotic lesion progression. On the other hand, post hoc analyses of data from 4S and WOSCOPS (see below) did not show reduction in TG to contribute to CHD risk reduction, whereas in CARE (see below) TG concentration during follow-up was only weakly associated with coronary event rate (Pedersen et al. *Circulation* 1998;97:1453–1460; West of Scotland Coronary Prevention Study Group *Circulation* 1998;97:1440–1445; Sacks et al. *Circulation* 1998;97:1446–1452). Baseline fasting TG values in these three statin trials were similar (133, 163, and 155 mg/dL, or 1.5, 1.8, and 1.7 mmol/L) despite fairly different enrollment criteria (≤220, <530, and <350 mg/dL, or ≤2.5, <6.0, and <4.0 mmol/L). In these analyses, change in HDL-C was found to contribute to the reduction in risk only in 4S, although the risk relation was not as strong as for TC, LDL-C, non-HDL-C, and apo B in that study.

It may not be possible to design a true TG-lowering trial because available TG-lowering drugs affect multiple lipoprotein families. However, data from trials targeting lipid fractions other than LDL-C are beginning to emerge. In the angiographic **Bezafibrate Coronary Atherosclerosis Intervention Trial** (BECAIT), conducted in young MI survivors with TC ≥200 mg/dL (≥5.2 mmol/L) and/or TG ≥140 mg/dL (≥1.6 mmol/L), fibrate use despite no significant change in LDL-C (treatment effect of -2%) was associated with significantly slowed progression of focal coronary atherosclerosis as well as a significantly reduced coronary event rate compared with placebo. Other lipid effects of bezafibrate in BECAIT included 35% and 31% reductions in VLDL-C and fasting TG and a 9% increase in HDL-C. Plasma fibrinogen was reduced 12% (Ericsson et al. *Lancet* 1996;347:849–853). On the basis of an unpublished, preliminary report, results of the **Bezafibrate Infarction Prevention** (BIP) study appear to be more equivocal. BIP was designed to assess the clinical coronary effects of lowering TG and increasing HDL-C in men and women with CHD and LDL-C ≤180 mg/dL (≤4.7 mmol/L), HDL-C ≤45 mg/dL (≤1.2 mmol/L), and TG ≤300 (≤3.4 mmol/L). Overall, there was no significant benefit with therapy in the primary endpoint of MI or sudden death (9% reduction), although that endpoint was significantly reduced (by 40%) in the subset of patients with baseline TG ≥200 mg/dL (≥2.3 mmol/L). Therapy lowered TG by 22% and fibrinogen by 9% and raised HDL-C by 12%, but reduced LDL-C by only 5%.

1.3.4 TC:HDL-C and LDL-C:HDL-C Ratios

The TC:HDL-C ratio was found to be a better predictor of CHD events than TC, LDL-C, HDL-C, or TG in the **Framingham Study** and several other studies. In 4-year Framingham data, individuals with TC <200 mg/dL (<5.2 mmol/L) but HDL-C <40 mg/dL (<1.0 mmol/L) had the same high risk as individuals with TC of 260 mg/dL (6.7 mmol/L), although HDL-C of 50–59 mg/dL (1.3–1.5 mmol/L) did not protect against TC of 260 mg/dL (Castelli *Atherosclerosis* 1996;124[suppl]:S1–S9). The TC:HDL-C ratio implicitly incorporates information on both LDL-C and TG in the numerator. In the **Münster Heart Study** (PROCAM) at 8-year follow-up, the number of observed definite CHD events per 1,000 subjects showed a curvilinear increase with increasing TC:HDL-C ratio, with a steep increase at a ratio of 5 (Figure 1.3-2). In the same study, an LDL-C:HDL-C ratio of 4–4.9 was associated with 64 observed events per 1,000 men, compared with only 18 events for a ratio <3. Events jumped to 171 per 1,000 for a ratio of 5–5.9, and to 278 for a ratio ≥7 (Assmann et al. *Eur Heart J* 1998;19[suppl A]:A2–A11).

1.3.5 The Lipid Triad

It appears that high risk for CHD is conferred when elevated TG and low HDL-C occur with elevated TC or LDL-C, or the TC:HDL-C or LDL-C:HDL-C ratio is high and TG is elevated. The cluster of lipid abnormalities identifies a patient group at high risk. In the **Münster Heart Study** (PROCAM) at 8-year follow-up of middle-aged men with no history of MI or cerebrovascular accident, fully one fourth of the CHD events occurred in the 4.3% of men who had plasma TG >200 mg/dL (>2.3 mmol/L) and an LDL-C:HDL-C ratio >5 (Assmann et al. *Am J Cardiol* 1996;77:1179–1184). The Münster results are highly concordant with post hoc analyses of the Helsinki Heart Study (see below).

1.3.6 Low HDL-C and Elevated TG

Evidence has also emerged from the **Framingham Study** (Castelli *Am Heart J* 1986;112:432–437) and other studies that the occurrence of low HDL-C in conjunction with elevated TG, even without or with only minor elevation of LDL-C, may confer increased risk for CHD. In the **Copenhagen Male Study**, conducted among men free of CVD at baseline, the combination of elevated TG and low HDL-C was at least as strong a predictor of CHD events as elevated LDL-C (highest fifth). Age-adjusted incidences of CHD during 8 years of follow-up were 11.4% and 8.2%, respectively (Jeppesen et al. *Arterioscler Thromb Vasc Biol* 1997;17:1114–1120). Thus, there may be an important high-risk group that would be overlooked were TG and HDL-C not measured.

The conjunction of low HDL-C and elevated TG representing VLDL-TG has been associated with resistance to insulin-stimulated glucose uptake,

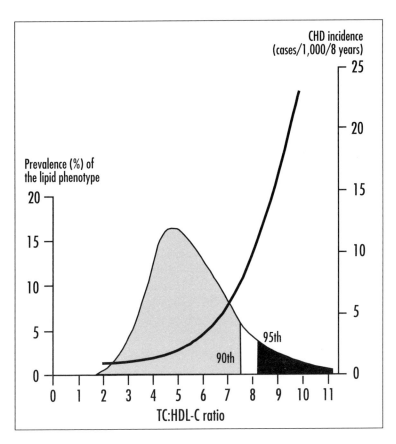

Figure 1.3-2. Risk for CHD according to TC:HDL-C ratio in the Münster Heart Study (PROCAM), 8-year follow-up. From The International Task Force for Prevention of Coronary Heart Disease. Coronary heart disease: Reducing the risk. The scientific background for primary and secondary prevention of coronary heart disease. *Nutr Metab Cardiovasc Dis* 1998;8:205–271; used with permission.

glucose intolerance, compensatory hyperinsulinemia, hypertension, higher uric acid concentrations, microalbuminuria, a procoagulant state (e.g., increased circulating concentrations of fibrinogen and plasminogen activator inhibitor 1), and the finding of small, dense LDL. The constellation is commonly referred to as the *cardiovascular metabolic syndrome, insulin resistance syndrome* (to highlight a leading proposed etiology), or *metabolic syndrome X* (one of the earliest names used). No causal relation has been established between insulin resistance and any of the problems, but regardless of whether insulin resistance itself predisposes to CHD or gives rise to the other components, many of the clustered factors are associated with risk for atherosclerosis and/or thrombosis. There is some evidence that the syndrome could originate in a generalized imbalance in the metabolism of carbohydrate and lipids. Contributing factors include obesity (especially abdominal obesity), diet (high intake of saturated fatty acids, excess calories), physical inactivity, aging, and genetic factors. Increased LDL-C is not part of the definition, and the clustered metabolic disturbances may help explain how CHD develops in the absence of hypercholesterolemia, at least as defined by current clinical action limits.

The cardiovascular metabolic syndrome appears to have a kinship with familial combined hyperlipidemia (whose fundamental basis remains to be elucidated), hyperapobetalipoproteinemia (hyper–apo B), or LDL phenotype B (a preponderance of small, dense LDL in plasma, associated in some studies with increased risk for MI). The low HDL-C and small, dense LDL, which together with elevated plasma TG are the "atherogenic dyslipidemia" of the syndrome, may arise in fact from an increased TG content of TG-rich lipoproteins. (See Figure E.1-3.)

When accomplished, weight loss and aerobic exercise are the most effective treatment for the metabolic and hemodynamic disturbances of the cardiovascular metabolic syndrome. Patients with this constellation of risk factors must be taught that lifestyle changes are of the utmost importance to their management.

1.4 Clinical Endpoint Trials of Cholesterol-Lowering Diets

A diet low in saturated fat and cholesterol is the key lifestyle change for decreasing LDL-C, although a high-carbohydrate diet may increase TG in sensitive individuals. Response to dietary modification is highly variable and is genetically influenced: some patients show dramatic lipid improvements, whereas others respond only minimally. Enough studies of compliance with dietary regimens have shown positive results to lead to the conclusion that meaningful dietary modification is possible. Weight loss and increased physical activity may moderately reduce LDL-C, but their chief effects are to increase HDL-C and decrease, sometimes markedly, elevated plasma TG. With smoking cessation, HDL-C rises and some studies have shown slight decreases in LDL-C.

A number of studies of cholesterol lowering by dietary therapy have been carried out. In the 5-year, nonblinded, randomized **Oslo Diet–Heart Study**, recurrent MI rate was significantly reduced 33% and CHD death rate was nonsignificantly reduced 26% in MI survivors given a low-fat, low-cholesterol diet (yielding a mean reduction in TC of 14%) rather than usual diet (Leren *Acta Med Scand Suppl* 1966;466:1–92). The **Los Angeles Veterans Administration Study**, which enrolled men both with and without CHD who were living in a veterans' home, used a 40%-fat diet; the experimental diet contained three times more polyunsaturated fat and 40% less cholesterol than the control diet. The experimental diet yielded a trend toward a reduction in the primary endpoint of acute MI or sudden cardiac death, and a significant risk reduction of 31% when the primary endpoint and other atherosclerotic events were pooled (Dayton et al. *Circulation* 1969;40[suppl II]:1–63). Cost and other considerations have prohibited definitive diet–heart trials in free-living subjects, given the lower degree of cholesterol reduction generally achieved with diet compared with drug therapy. Perhaps 10% of the population at large is diet resistant. Nevertheless, dietary modification is the cornerstone of lipid management and can play an important role in lowering cholesterol concentrations and reducing CHD death and disability in the world.

1.5 Clinical Endpoint Trials of Cholesterol-Lowering Drugs

1.5.1 Primary-Prevention Trials

Early pharmacologic clinical trial efforts to reduce first CHD events through cholesterol lowering were successful despite relatively small decreases in LDL-C. Both the **Lipid Research Clinics Coronary Primary**

Prevention Trial (LRC-CPPT) and the **Helsinki Heart Study** enrolled hypercholesterolemic middle-aged men (mean baseline LDL-C values of 204 and 188 mg/dL, or 5.3 and 4.9 mmol/L). In the LRC-CPPT, therapy with cholestyramine reduced TC and LDL-C 8% and 13% more than placebo, and with an average time on trial of 7 years, the rate of CHD death and/or nonfatal MI was a significant 19% lower in the drug group. The trial's results confirmed the 2:1 ratio between CHD risk reduction and cholesterol lowering predicted by observational epidemiologic studies and spurred development of the first adult clinical guidelines of the NCEP. Efficacy was limited by the resin's poor tolerability, related in chief to GI complaints (Lipid Research Clinics Program *JAMA* 1984;251:351–364, 365–374). In the Helsinki Heart Study, 5 years of treatment with gemfibrozil significantly reduced CHD incidence (cardiac death plus MI) by 34%; lipid changes compared with placebo included an 11% reduction in LDL-C, 35% reduction in fasting TG, and 11% increase in HDL-C (Frick et al. *N Engl J Med* 1987;317:1237–1245). Post hoc analyses of the Helsinki data have narrowed greatest CHD benefit to patients with an LDL-C:HDL-C ratio >5 and TG >200 mg/dL (>2.3 mmol/L) (71% risk reduction) (Manninen et al. *Circulation* 1992; 85:37–45) and more specifically to overweight patients, who often had multiple risk factors (78% risk reduction) (Tenkanen et al. *Circulation* 1995;92:1779–1785).

Although these trials were not designed to assess effects of intervention on all-cause mortality rate, the absence of survival benefit led some investigators to question the value of cholesterol-lowering drug therapy in patients without known CHD. With the availability of the statins, the question of whether cholesterol lowering is beneficial has been very clearly resolved (Tables 1.5-1 and 1.5-2). The 5-year **West of Scotland Coronary Prevention Study** (WOSCOPS) evaluated pravastatin 40 mg/day or placebo in 6,595 hypercholesterolemic, high-risk middle-aged men with no history of MI (although small percentages had a history of angina pectoris or intermittent claudication). Mean baseline LDL-C was 192 mg/dL (5.0 mmol/L). With a 26% reduction in LDL-C (to a mean 159 mg/dL, or 4.1 mmol/L), statin therapy doubled the efficacy of cholesterol lowering seen in earlier trials, and it achieved substantial reductions in both CHD event rates (31% in CHD death or nonfatal MI and 37% in need for CABG

Table 1.5-1. Effect of HMG-CoA Reductase Inhibitor Therapy on Ischemic Events: Clinical Event Trials

Trial and Agent	Baseline LDL-C, mg/dL (mmol/L)	↓LDL-C	LDL-C Achieved, mg/dL (mmol/L)	Event(s)	Follow-up, yr	Statin Event Rate	Placebo Event Rate	RRR	ARR*	NNT†
Primary prevention										
WOSCOPS,‡ pravastatin	192 (5.0)	26%§	159 (4.1)	Nonfatal MI or CHD death	4.9	174/3,302 5.3%	248/3,293 7.5%	31%	2.2%	45
AFCAPS/ TexCAPS, lovastatin	150 (3.9)	25%‖	115 (3.0)‖	Nonfatal or fatal MI, unstable angina, or sudden cardiac death as first event	5.2	116/3,304 3.5%	183/3,301 5.5%	37%	2.0%	50
Secondary prevention										
4S,¶ simvastatin	188 (4.9)	35%	122 (3.2)	All-cause death (primary endpoint)	5.4	182/2,221 8.2%	256/2,223 11.5%	30%	3.3%	30
				Nonfatal MI, coronary death, or resuscitated cardiac arrest		431/2,221 19.4%	622/2,223 27.9%	34%	8.5%	12
CARE,¶ pravastatin	139 (3.6)	32%#	98 (2.5)	Nonfatal MI or CHD death	5.0	212/2,081 10.2%	274/2,078 13.2%	24%	3.0%	33
LIPID,‡ pravastatin	150 (3.9) median	25%**	112 (2.9)	Nonfatal MI or CHD death	6.1	557/4,512 12.3%	715/4,502 15.9%	24%	3.6%	28
AVERT, atorvastatin	145 (3.7)††	46%	77 (2.0)	Ischemic events (death, non-fatal MI, cerebrovascular accident, CABG, PTCA, worsening angina with hospitalization)	1.5	11/164 6.7%	Angioplasty + usual care‡‡ 25/177 14.1%	36%	7.4%	14

Source: Modified from Jacobson TA, Schein JR, Williamson A, et al. Maximizing the cost-effectiveness of lipid-lowering therapy. *Arch Intern Med* 1998;158:1977–1989; used with permission. Copyright 1998, American Medical Association.

Note: ARR = absolute risk reduction; NNT = number needed to treat; RRR = relative risk reduction.

*ARR was calculated as the placebo event rate minus the statin event rate.
†See also Appendix D.9.3.
‡By number of events.
§In patients actually treated; LDL–C reduction was 17% in all patients randomized to pravastatin.
‖At 1 year.
¶By number of patients.
#Reduction from baseline; 28% reduction compared with placebo.
**Percentage average difference between pravastatin and placebo.
††Without a washout period from previous lipid-lowering medication; at randomization, 26% of patients were taking lipid-lowering medication in the atorvastatin group.
‡‡Patients recommended for angioplasty were randomized to atorvastatin plus usual medical therapy, or to angioplasty plus usual care (which included lipid-lowering pharmacotherapy in 73%).

Table 1.5-2. Additional Key Points of HMG-CoA Reductase Inhibitor Clinical Event Trials

Trial	Year Pub.	Sex and Age, yr	Agent and Daily Dose, mg	Enrollment Lipids, mg/dL (mmol/L)	Key Clinical Effects and p Values	
Primary prevention						
WOSCOPS*	1995	M, 45–64	Pravastatin, 40	LDL-C ≥155 (≥4.0) TG ≤530 (≤6.0)	• Coronary events ↓31%	<0.001
					• No excess non-CVD death	
					• Total mortality ↓22%	0.051
					• CABG or PTCA ↓37%	0.009
AFCAPS/ TexCAPS*	1998	M, 45–73 F, 55–73	Lovastatin, 20–40	TC 180–264 (4.7–6.8) LDL-C 130–190 (3.4–4.9) HDL-C ≤45 (≤1.16) M, ≤47 (≤1.22) F TG ≤400 (≤4.5)	• Coronary events ↓37%, including unstable angina	<0.001
					• No excess non-CVD death	
					• CABG or PTCA ↓33%	0.001
Secondary prevention						
4S	1994	M/F, 35–70	Simvastatin, 20–40	TC 212–309 (5.5–8.0) TG ≤220 (≤2.5)	• Total mortality ↓30%	<0.001
					• Coronary events ↓34%	<0.001
					• CABG or PTCA ↓37%	<0.001
					• Post hoc: Stroke or TIA ↓30%	0.024
CARE	1996	M/F, 21–75	Pravastatin, 40	TC <240 (<6.2) LDL-C 115–174 (3.0–4.5) TG <350 (<4.0)	• Coronary events ↓24%	0.003
					• No excess non-CVD death	
					• Stroke ↓32%	0.03
					• CABG or PTCA ↓27%	<0.001
LIPID	1998	M/F, 31–75	Pravastatin, 40	TC 155–270 (4.0–7.0) TG ≤445 (≤5.0)	• Coronary events ↓24%	<0.001
					• Coronary death ↓24%	<0.001
					• Total mortality ↓22%	<0.001
					• Stroke ↓19%	0.048
					• CABG or PTCA ↓20%	<0.001
AVERT	1999	M/F, 18–80 (mean 59)	Atorvastatin, 80	LDL-C ≥115 (≥3.0) TG ≤500 (≤5.6)	• Ischemic events ↓36%	0.048†
					• Decreased time to first ischemic event	0.027

Note: See text for full names of trials.
*In WOSCOPS, 77% of patients would have been drug eligible by 1993 NCEP adult guidelines. In AFCAPS/TexCAPS, 17% would have been drug eligible.
†Versus an adjusted significance level of p = 0.045.

or PTCA) and all-cause mortality rate (22%). Treatment also lowered TG by 12% and increased HDL-C by 5% (Shepherd et al. *N Engl J Med* 1995;333:1301–1307).

Similar lipid changes (LDL-C -25%, TG -15%, HDL-C +6%) and CHD risk reduction (unstable angina, MI, and sudden cardiac death -37%, coronary revascularization -33%) were achieved with the 20–40 mg/day lovastatin used in the 5-year **Air Force/Texas Coronary Atherosclerosis Prevention Study** (AFCAPS/TexCAPS) (Downs et al. *JAMA* 1998;279:1615–1622). AFCAPS/TexCAPS, however, differed from previous primary-prevention trials of cholesterol-lowering pharmacotherapy in enrolling, in addition to middle-aged men, both (postmenopausal) women and elderly patients (aged 65–73); moreover, the patients had only average cholesterol concentrations (mean baseline TC and LDL-C of 221 and 150 mg/dL, or 5.7 and 3.9 mmol/L) and below-average HDL-C (36 mg/dL in men and 40 mg/dL in women, or 0.9 and 1.0 mmol/L). Mean LDL-C achieved with statin therapy was 115 mg/dL (3.0 mmol/L). The trial was a very pure test of primary prevention: the 6,605 subjects had no history, signs, or symptoms of definite MI, angina, cerebrovascular accident, TIA, or claudication. Treatment benefit on first major coronary event (fatal or nonfatal MI, unstable angina, or sudden cardiac death) applied equally to both younger and older patients, and although the number of events was small, CHD incidence was reduced 46% among women in the drug group compared with women in the placebo group. Benefit was seen as well in other predefined subgroups such as hypertensive patients and smokers—that is, statin therapy appears to attenuate the CHD risk conferred by a number of other major risk factors, so that the higher the baseline risk, the greater the absolute benefit with treatment.

Whereas in nonstatin clinical endpoint trials, it appeared that about 2 years of cholesterol-lowering therapy was required for benefit, in both WOSCOPS and AFCAPS/TexCAPS a divergence between the drug and placebo groups in CHD events began to emerge <1 year after the beginning of therapy (Figure 1.5-1). Seventy-seven percent of WOSCOPS subjects would have fallen within current NCEP categories for consideration of drug therapy, and in WOSCOPS cost per life-year saved compared favorably with smoking cessation programs, exercise programs, antihypertension medications, CABG, PTCA, and other interventions widely used in CHD prevention. This economic analysis is in accord with a number of studies that have shown statin therapy to be cost effective in high-risk subsets of primary-prevention patients (see D.9). In AFCAPS/TexCAPS, on the other hand, only 17% of the patients would have been eligible for lipid-lowering drug therapy according to current NCEP guidelines. The study's findings would support benefit of statin treatment in about 6 million Americans currently outside NCEP drug eligibility criteria; whether that benefit is considered affordable is largely a political matter.

1.5.2 Secondary-Prevention Trials

Results of clinical endpoint trials leave no doubt that elevated LDL-C must be lowered in patients with established atherosclerotic disease. A variety of studies have found lipid-lowering therapy, including statin therapy, to be cost effective in almost all secondary-prevention patients (see D.9).

Meta-analysis of nonstatin secondary-prevention trials found a 10% reduction in TC to yield 19%, 12%, and 15% reductions in rates of nonfatal, fatal, and all MIs (Rossouw et al. *N Engl J Med* 1990;323:1112–1119). In the 6-year **Coronary Drug Project** (CDP), several interventions were compared with placebo in 8,341 men with a history of at least one MI. The estrogen and dextrothyroxine arms of the trial were discontinued early because of either increased mortality or side effects, and there was no clinical benefit with clofibrate therapy. But the group receiving nicotinic acid showed a 10% reduction in TC and a decrease in nonfatal MI rate (Coronary Drug Project Study Group *JAMA* 1975;231:360–381). In mortality follow-up 9 years after intervention ended, all-cause mortality was significantly reduced 11% in the nicotinic acid group (Canner et al. *J Am Coll Cardiol* 1986;8:1245–1255). The **Stockholm Ischemic Heart Disease Secondary Prevention Study** randomized 555 male and female MI survivors to combination therapy with clofibrate and nicotinic acid or to a control group. After 5 years, significant changes in the drug group included reductions in TC (13%), fasting TG (19%), CHD death rate (36%), and total mortality rate (26%). Retrospective subset analysis showed the decrease in CHD mortality to be directly related to the decrease in TG (Carlson and Rosenhamer *Acta Med Scand* 1988;223:405–418).

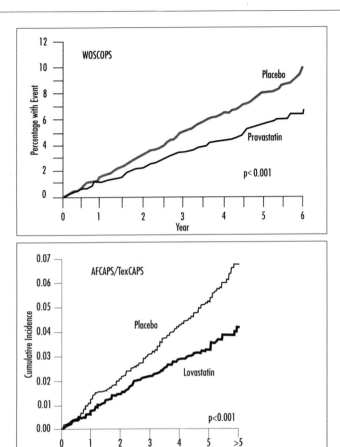

Figure 1.5-1. Time to first definite coronary event (primary endpoint) in high- and lower-risk patients randomized to statin therapy or placebo in primary preven- tion. The high-risk patients of the West of Scotland Coronary Prevention Study (WOSCOPS) had a mean baseline LDL-C concentration of 192 mg/dL (5.0 mmol/L); at the average follow-up of 4.9 years, the primary endpoint of nonfatal MI or CHD death was significantly reduced by 31% with pravastatin therapy. Extension of benefit to gen- erally healthy patients with only average cholesterol concentrations was achieved in the Air Force/Texas Coronary Atherosclerosis Prevention Study (AFCAPS/TexCAPS), in which relative risk for the composite primary endpoint of fatal or nonfatal MI, sudden death, or unstable angina was significantly lowered by 37% in the lovastatin group at the average follow-up of 5.2 years. Mean baseline LDL-C in AFCAPS/TexCAPS was 150 mg/dL (3.9 mmol/L); in addition, AFCAPS/TexCAPS patients had decreased HDL-C at baseline: a mean 36 mg/dL (0.94 mmol/L) in men and 40 mg/dL (1.03 mmol/L) in women. From Shepherd J, Cobbe SM, Ford I, et al., for the West of Scotland Coronary Prevention Study Group. Prevention of coronary heart disease with pravastatin in men with hypercholesterolemia. *N Engl J Med* 1995;333:1301–1307, and Downs JR, Clearfield M, Weis S, et al. Primary prevention of acute coronary events with lovastatin in men and women with average cholesterol levels. Results of AFCAPS/TexCAPS. *JAMA* 1998;279:1615–1622; used with permission.

Publication of the results of large, long-term trials of statins with clinical endpoints (Tables 1.5-1 and 1.5-2) removed any doubts about the value of cholesterol-lowering therapy in patients with established CHD, in particular because of the achievement of unequivocal survival benefit. The **Scandinavian Simvastatin Survival Study** (4S, testing simvastatin 20–40 mg/day), **Cholesterol and Recurrent Events** (CARE) trial (pravastatin 40 mg/day), and **Long-term Intervention with Pravastatin in Ischemic Disease** (LIPID) trial (pravastatin 40 mg/day) together enrolled nearly 18,000 men and women with a history of MI and/or angina pectoris. The findings of the 5–6 years of intervention in the trials were remarkably concordant (Scandinavian Simvastatin Survival Study Group *Lancet* 1994;344:1383–1389; Sacks et al. *N Engl J Med* 1996;335:1001–1009; Long-term Intervention with Pravastatin in Ischaemic Disease Study Group *N Engl J Med* 1998;339:1349–1357). Baseline LDL-C concentrations represented a wide spectrum of values— from the upper tail of the western population distribution in 4S (mean 188 mg/dL, or 4.9 mmol/L) to only average values in CARE (median 139 mg/dL, or 3.6 mmol/L), and a broad range in the 9,014 patients of LIPID (median 150 mg/dL, or 3.9 mmol/L; enrollment TC 155–270 mg/dL, or 4.0–7.0 mmol/L). Statin therapy reduced LDL-C by 25–35%, to 122, 98, and 112 mg/dL (3.2, 2.5, and 2.9 mmol/L) in the respective trials. Fasting TG was decreased by 10–14% and HDL-C was increased by 5–8%. The sole primary endpoint in 4S was total mortality rate, which was highly significantly reduced by 30% compared with placebo, a result confirmed by the significant 22% reduction of all-cause mortality as a secondary endpoint in LIPID. In each of the three trials therapy was safe and well tolerated; in none was there any excess of non-CVD mortality. The rate of major coronary events was reduced by 24–34%, with need for coronary revascularization reduced by 20–37%. Coronary benefit extended to women, the elderly (ages at enrollment ranging to 75 years), and diabetic patients as subpopulations in the trials. Combined analysis of results from WOSCOPS, CARE, and LIPID in the **Prospective Pravastatin Pooling Project** showed significant, consistent reductions in coronary event rates in elderly (-26%) and nonelderly (-22%) patients, men (-23%) and women (-27%), and diabetic (-26%) and nondiabetic (-23%) patients (Sacks et al. *Circulation* 1999;100[suppl I]:I-238–I-239 [abstract 1238]). In

4S benefit began after about 1 year of therapy and increased steadily thereafter; in CARE and LIPID a clear difference occurred from 2 years' follow-up. Meta-analysis of 13 statin trials and 46 trials of other cholesterol-lowering interventions found that variability in mortality results across the trials could largely be explained by differences in the magnitude of cholesterol lowering. Only statins as a class in this analysis showed large and statistically significant reductions in CHD death rate (-34%) and all-cause mortality rate (-25%) (Bucher et al. *Arterioscler Thromb Vasc Biol* 1999;19:187–195).

An unexpected finding in these statin trials was a reduction in risk for cerebrovascular events. Stroke risk as a prespecified endpoint was decreased by 32% in CARE and by 19% in LIPID, and post hoc analyses showed risk for stroke or TIA to be reduced by 30% in 4S and by 27% in CARE, all differences statistically significant (Plehn et al. *Circulation* 1999;99:216–223; Long-term Intervention with Pravastatin in Ischaemic Disease Study Group *N Engl J Med* 1998;339:1349–1357; Scandinavian Simvastatin Survival Study Group *Lancet* 1994;344:1383–1389). There was no increase in risk for hemorrhagic stroke. The stroke benefit has been corroborated by several retrospective meta-analyses of a variety of statin trials; the 24–31% risk reduction described by meta-analysis suggests an effect similar to that of aspirin in secondary prevention (Delanty and Vaughan *Stroke* 1997;28:2315–2320). The stroke benefit is supported by imaging studies that have shown improvement in carotid atherosclerosis with statin therapy (e.g., Furberg et al. *Circulation* 1994;90:1679–1687; MacMahon et al. *Circulation* 1998;97:1784–1790). Because evidence relating plasma cholesterol and stroke has been equivocal, it has been suggested that the statins' apparent efficacy against cerebrovascular disease may lie in an effect of stabilizing atherosclerotic lesions (the concept of lesion stabilization is discussed in Appendix E.2.4). The result could also be related to the statins' greater cholesterol-lowering potency. Cerebrovascular event reduction was also seen, however, in HIT, in which LDL-C concentration was not significantly affected by therapy (see 1.3.2). Patients in HIT's gemfibrozil group had a 25% lower relative risk for confirmed stroke (p = 0.10) and a 59% lower risk for TIA (p <0.001) (Rubins et al. *N Engl J Med* 1999;341:410–418). Beyond gemfibrozil's improvement of HDL-C and TG concentrations, and perhaps other aspects of the cardiovascular metabolic syndrome, fibrates have well-known beneficial effects on a number of coagulation and fibrinolytic factors.

The shorter-term (18-month) **Atorvastatin Versus Revascularization Treatments** (AVERT) trial compared atorvastatin 80 mg/day with angioplasty and usual care in 341 angioplasty-eligible patients with stable CHD. Atorvastatin therapy, which was well tolerated, reduced LDL-C by 46%, from a mean value at randomization (without a washout period from previous lipid-lowering medication) of 145 mg/dL (3.7 mmol/L) to 77 mg/dL (2.0 mmol/L), as well as decreased plasma TG by 11% and increased HDL-C by 8%. Lipid changes with usual care in the angioplasty group included an 18% decrease in LDL-C (from 147 to 119 mg/dL, or from 3.8 to 3.1 mmol/L), a 10% increase in TG, and an 11% increase in HDL-C; 73% of patients in this group were receiving lipid-lowering drug therapy. The rate of ischemic events (death, nonfatal MI, cerebrovascular accident, CABG, angioplasty, worsening angina resulting in hospitalization) was reduced by 36% (p = 0.048 vs. an adjusted significance level of p = 0.045) in the patients with aggressive reduction of LDL-C with atorvastatin. In addition, the time to first ischemic event was significantly reduced in the atorvastatin group (Pitt et al. *N Engl J Med* 1999;341:70–76). Post hoc analysis showed that significantly fewer ischemic events occurred in patients with LDL-C reduction >40% compared with those with reduction <40%. But while meta-analysis, as noted above, has indicated that the CHD and total mortality risk reductions with statins can be attributed to their cholesterol-lowering effect and appear to be largely related to the degree to which they lower cholesterol (Gould et al. *Circulation* 1998;97:946–952; Bucher et al. *Arterioscler Thromb Vasc Biol* 1999;19:187–195), data are needed from randomized clinical trials designed to test formally whether "lower is better." The question is being addressed in secondary prevention by the 5-year **Treating to New Targets** (TNT) trial (Figure 1.5-2), using two dosages of atorvastatin (10 and 80 mg/day); by the 5.5-year **Incremental Decrease in Endpoints through Aggressive Lipid Lowering** (IDEAL) trial, using atorvastatin (80 mg/day) and simvastatin (20–40 mg/day); and by the 4-month **Myocardial Ischemia Reduction with Aggressive Cholesterol Lowering** (MIRACL) study, using atorvastatin (80 mg/day). Until results are available, the ILIB recommends that guidelines aiming for LDL-C below 100 mg/dL (2.6 mmol/L) should be followed.

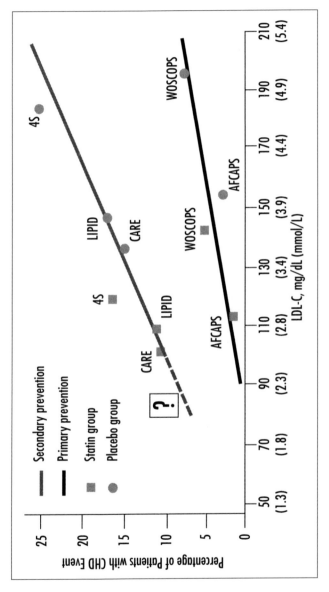

Figure 1.5-2. Hypothesis of the Treating to New Targets (TNT) trial. The ongoing secondary-prevention TNT trial is directly examining whether "lower is better" in cholesterol lowering to reduce CHD events. Patients with initial LDL-C 130–230 mg/dL (3.4–5.9 mmol/L) and TG ≤600 mg/dL (≤6.8 mmol/L) who achieve LDL-C <130 mg/dL (<3.4 mmol/L) after 8 weeks of diet and atorvastatin 10 mg/day are randomized to double-blind therapy with atorvastatin 10 or 80 mg/day (respective targets, ≤100 and ≤75 mg/dL, or ≤2.6 and ≤1.9 mmol/L). WOSCOPS, CARE, and LIPID tested pravastatin, 4S simvastatin, and AFCAPS/TexCAPS lovastatin as cholesterol-lowering therapy (see text for full names of trials). Modified from Kastelein JJP. The future of best practice. *Atherosclerosis* 1999;143(suppl 1):S17–S21; used with permission.

Table 1.6-1. Representative Lipid-Modifying Trials Assessing Coronary Atherosclerosis by Angiography

Trial	Baseline LDL-C in Treatment Group	Intervention	% LDL-C Decrease vs. Baseline	% Patients with Progression, Treatment/ Control	Clinical Events, Treatment/ Control
STARS	193 (5.0)	Diet alone	-16	15/46	3/10*
	203 (5.2)	Cholestyramine	-36	12/46	1/10*
CCAIT	173 (4.5)	Lovastatin	-29	33/50	15/20
REGRESS	166 (4.3)	Pravastatin	-25	56/69	10/17*
BECAIT	180 (4.7)	Bezafibrate	-4 †	74/85	3/11*
LOCAT	139 (3.6)	Gemfibrozil	-5 ‡	—	7/7
Post-CABG	155 (4.0)	Aggressive vs. moderate lovastatin	-37 to -40 vs. -13 to -15	27 vs. 39 (% of grafts)	85 vs. 103
LCAS	146 (3.8)	Fluvastatin	-24	29/39	31/41
FATS	196 (5.1)	Lovastatin + colestipol	-46	21/46	3/10*
	190 (4.9)	Niacin + colestipol	-32	25/46	2/10*
POSCH	179 (4.6)	Partial ileal bypass	-42	38/65	82/125*

Note: **BECAIT** = Bezafibrate Coronary Atherosclerosis Intervention Trial—Ericsson et al. *Lancet* 1996;347:849–853; **CCAIT** = Canadian Coronary Atherosclerosis Intervention Trial—Waters et al. *Circulation* 1994;89:959–968; **FATS** = Familial Atherosclerosis Treatment Study—Brown et al. *N Engl J Med* 1990;323:1289–1298; **LCAS** = Lipoprotein and Coronary Atherosclerosis Study—Herd et al. *Am J Cardiol* 1997;80:278–286; **LOCAT** = Lopid Coronary Angiography Trial—Frick et al. *Circulation* 1997;96:2137–2143; **POSCH** = Program on the Surgical Control of the Hyperlipidemias—Buchwald et al. *N Engl J Med* 1990;323:946–955; **Post-CABG** = Post Coronary Artery Bypass Graft Trial—Post Coronary Artery Bypass Graft Trial Investigators *N Engl J Med* 1997;336:153–162; **REGRESS** = Regression Growth Evaluation Statin Study—Jukema et al. *Circulation* 1995;91:2528–2540; **STARS** = St. Thomas' Atherosclerosis Regression Study—Watts et al. *Lancet* 1992;339:563–569.

*Statistically significant difference.

†The principal lipid changes in BECAIT were a 31% decrease in fasting TG and a 9% increase in HDL-C. In addition, plasma fibrinogen decreased 12% with treatment.

‡The principal lipid changes in LOCAT were a 40% decrease in fasting TG and a 9% increase in HDL-C (medians).

1.6 Imaging Trials

Angiographic monitoring has provided another approach to assessing effects of lipid-regulating therapy on coronary atherosclerotic disease. The results of more than 20 such trials, which typically enrolled relatively small numbers of patients and which lasted 1–5 years, have been reported; representative trials are described in Table 1.6-1. On the whole, the angiographic trials, using a variety of drug and lifestyle interventions and even surgery, demonstrated that intensive lipid modification retards the progression and, in a small subset of patients, leads to the regression of coronary atherosclerosis. Significant reductions in the formation of new lesions occurred as well. Benefit in women in the trials that included a sufficient proportion of women to enable subset analysis was similar to that in men. The angiographic benefit of pharmacologic lipid lowering was confirmed by trials using B-mode ultrasound to monitor carotid atherosclerosis, which is a risk marker for both CHD and stroke.

Nearly all the angiographic trials tested cholesterol lowering, and lesion benefit was seen across a wide range of baseline LDL-C values. However, significant retardation of coronary lesion progression was also achieved, as noted in earlier sections, in BECAIT and LOCAT with therapies targeting in chief lipid fractions other than LDL-C and with little or no LDL-C reduction achieved. On the other hand, in the **Post Coronary Artery Bypass Graft** (Post-CABG) trial, which assessed the effects of cholesterol lowering on saphenous vein grafts, the patients who had LDL-C lowered to a range of 93 to 97 mg/dL (2.4–2.5 mmol/L) by aggressive lovastatin treatment did significantly better than those who achieved LDL-C in the range of 132 to 136 mg/dL (3.4–3.5 mmol/L) with moderate lovastatin treatment. Aggressive LDL-C reduction was associated not only with a significantly reduced risk for progression compared with moderate treatment but also with a 29% lower rate of revascularization procedures (Post Coronary Artery Bypass Graft Trial Investigators *N Engl J Med* 1997;336:153–162). Benefit against progression occurred irrespective of sex, age, and certain risk factors (smoking, hypertension, diabetes, and borderline high-risk triglyceride concentration) (Campeau et al. *Circulation* 1999;99:3241–3247).

Marked reductions of approximately 40–80% in acute coronary syndromes despite small, although statistically significant differences in angiographic change, typically in the range of 1% to 2% between the treatment and placebo groups (Kinlay et al. *Curr Opin Lipidol* 1996;7:389–397), were an unexpected finding in the imaging trials. A plausible hypothesis for the apparent discrepancy between the modest scale of stenosis benefit and the large clinical benefit in the trials is that lipid-regulating therapy may help stabilize atherosclerotic lesions. This thinking fits with the model developed from very careful pathologic analyses that most clinical events arise from angiographically mild or moderate lesions that are unstable and prone to rupture, as is described in Appendix E.2. Thus, the lipid-lowering regression trials may have helped set the stage for our new understanding of vascular biology and vessel wall dynamics.

1.7 Cholesterol Reduction and Endothelial Function

Endothelial function is impaired in atherosclerotic arteries, predisposing to inflammatory cell recruitment, vasoconstriction, and thrombosis. A number of randomized studies, including coronary studies, have demonstrated improvement in endothelium-mediated vasomotor function with cholesterol lowering by statins, resins, or LDL apheresis in patients with and without atherosclerotic disease (e.g., Egashira et al. *Circulation* 1994;89:2519–2524; Treasure et al. *N Engl J Med* 1995;332:481–487; Simons et al. *Atherosclerosis* 1998;137:197–203). Vasomotor function has usually been assessed by: quantitative coronary angiography, measuring changes after infusion of acetylcholine; ultrasonography, measuring changes in brachial artery diameter after induction of hyperemia by blood pressure cuff occlusion; and venous plethysmography, measuring forearm blood flow after intraarterial infusion of a cholinergic stimulus (e.g., methacholine). Improvement has usually been demonstrated within a few weeks of the initiation of therapy. It may be that anything that substantially lowers LDL (including oxidized LDL) may make arteries respond more like healthy arteries. Among other interventions that may have beneficial effects are smoking cessation, regular exercise, blood pressure lowering, ERT, and administration of 5-methyltetrahydrofolate, the active circulating form of folic acid.

1.8 SUGGESTED READING

1.8.1 General

Assmann G, Cullen P, Jossa F, et al., for the International Task Force for Prevention of Coronary Heart Disease. Coronary heart disease: Reducing the risk. The scientific background to primary and secondary prevention of coronary heart desease. A worldwide view. *Arterioscler Thromb Vasc Biol* 1999;19:1819–1824.

Davignon J, Genest J Jr. Genetics of lipoprotein disorders. *Endocrinol Metab Clin North Am* 1998;27:521–550.

Gotto AM Jr, Pownall HJ. *Manual of Lipid Disorders: Reducing the Risk for Coronary Heart Disease,* ed. 2. Baltimore: Williams and Wilkins, 1999.

The International Task Force for Prevention of Coronary Heart Disease. Coronary heart disease: Reducing the risk. The scientific background for primary and secondary prevention of coronary heart disease. A worldwide view. *Nutr Metab Cardiovasc Dis* 1998;8:205–271. Available at www.chd-taskforce.com.

Manson JE, Gaziano JM, Ridker PM, et al. Myocardial infarction: Epidemiologic overview. In: Manson JE, Ridker PM, Gaziano JM, et al., eds. *Prevention of Myocardial Infarction.* New York: Oxford University Press, 1996:3–31.

National Cholesterol Education Program. Second report of the Expert Panel on Detection, Evaluation, and Treatment of High Blood Cholesterol in Adults (Adult Treatment Panel II). *Circulation* 1994;89:1329–1445.

Prevention of coronary heart disease in clinical practice. Recommendations of the Second Joint Task Force of European and other Societies on Coronary Prevention. *Eur Heart J* 1998;19:1434–1503.

Rifai N, Warnick GR, Dominiczak MH, eds. *Handbook of Lipoprotein Testing,* ed. 2. Washington, DC: AACC Press, 2000. Available: American Association for Clinical Chemistry, telephone 202-857-0717.

Ryan TJ, Antman EM, Brooks NH, et al. ACC/AHA guidelines for the management of patients with acute myocardial infarction: 1999 update. Available at www.acc.org.

Scriver CR, Beaudet AL, Sly WS, et al., eds. *The Metabolic and Molecular Bases of Inherited Disease,* ed. 7, vol. 2. New York: McGraw-Hill, 1995:1841–2099.

Willett W. *Nutritional Epidemiology.* New York: Oxford University Press, 1990.

World Health Organization. *The World Health Report 1998.* Geneva: World Health Organization, 1998.

1.8.2 Multiple Risk Factors

Assmann G, Cullen P, Schulte H. The Münster Heart Study (PROCAM): Results of follow-up at 8 years. *Eur Heart J* 1998;19(suppl A):A2–A11.

Austin MA, Edwards KL. Small, dense low density lipoproteins, the insulin resistance syndrome and non-insulin-dependent diabetes. *Curr Opin Lipidol* 1996;7:167–171.

Gotto AM Jr, Lenfant C, Paoletti R, et al., eds. *Multiple Risk Factors in Cardiovascular Disease: Strategies of Prevention of Coronary Heart Disease, Cardiac Failure, and Stroke.* Dordrecht: Kluwer Academic, 1998:275–284.

Grundy SM, Balady GJ, Criqui MH, et al. Primary prevention of coronary heart disease: Guidance from Framingham. A statement for healthcare professionals from the AHA Task Force on Risk Reduction. *Circulation* 1998;97:1876–1887.

Grundy SM, Pasternack R, Greenland P, et al. Assessment of cardiovascular risk by use of multiple-risk-factor assessment equations. AHA/ACC scientific statement. *J Am Coll Cardiol* 1999;34:1348–1359.

Manninen V, Tenkanen L, Koskinen P, et al. Joint effects of serum triglyceride and LDL cholesterol and HDL cholesterol concentration on coronary heart disease risk in the Helsinki Heart Study: Implications for treatment. *Circulation* 1992;85:37–45.

Reaven GM. Pathophysiology of insulin resistance in human disease. *Physiol Rev* 1995;75:473–486.

Reaven GM, Laws A, eds. *Insulin Resistance: The Metabolic Syndrome X.* Totowa, NJ: Humana Press, 1999.

Wilson PWF, Kannel WB, Silbershatz H, et al. Clustering of metabolic factors and coronary heart disease. *Arch Intern Med* 1999;159:1104–1109.

Yusuf HR, Giles WH, Croft JB, et al. Impact of multiple risk factor profiles on determining cardiovascular disease risk. *Prev Med* 1998;27:1–9.

1.8.3 TC and LDL-C

Chen Z, Peto R, Collins R, et al. Serum cholesterol concentration and coronary heart disease in population with low cholesterol concentrations. *Br Med J* 1991;303:276–282.

Grundy SM. Role of low-density lipoproteins in atherogenesis and development of coronary heart disease. *Clin Chem* 1995;41:139–146.

Klag MJ, Ford DE, Mead LA, et al. Serum cholesterol in young men and subsequent cardiovascular disease. *N Engl J Med* 1993;328:313–318.

Law MR, Wald NJ, Thompson SG. Serum cholesterol reduction and health: By how much and how quickly is the risk of ischaemic heart disease lowered? *Br Med J* 1994;308:367–372.

1.8.4 HDL-C

Assmann G, Schulte H, von Eckardstein A, et al. High-density lipoprotein cholesterol as a predictor of coronary heart disease risk. The PROCAM experience and pathophysiological implications for reverse cholesterol transport. *Atherosclerosis* 1996;124(suppl):S11–S20.

Barter PJ, Rye K-A. High density lipoproteins and coronary heart disease. *Atherosclerosis* 1996;121:1–12.

Funke H. Genetic determinants of high-density lipoprotein levels. *Curr Opin Lipidol* 1997;8:189–196.

Gordon DJ. Factors affecting high-density lipoproteins. *Endocrinol Metab Clin North Am* 1998;27:699–709.

Gordon DJ, Probstfield JL, Garrison RJ, et al. High-density lipoprotein cholesterol and cardiovascular disease. Four prospective American studies. *Circulation* 1989;79:8–15.

Gotto AM Jr. Prognostic and therapeutic significance of low levels of high-density lipoprotein cholesterol. Current perspectives. *Arch Intern Med* 1999;159:1038–1040.

Harper CR, Jacobson TA. New perspectives on the management of low levels of high-density lipoprotein cholesterol. *Arch Intern Med* 1999;159:1049–1057.

Tailleux A, Fruchart JC. HDL heterogeneity and atherosclerosis. *Crit Rev Clin Lab Sci* 1996;33:163–201.

Vega GL, Grundy SM. Hypoalphalipoproteinemia (low high density lipoprotein) as a risk factor for coronary heart disease. *Curr Opin Lipidol* 1996;7:209–216.

1.8.5 Plasma TG

Assmann G, Schulte H, von Eckardstein A. Hypertriglyceridemia and elevated lipoprotein(a) are risk factors for major coronary events in middle-aged men. *Am J Cardiol* 1996;77:1179–1184.

Davignon J, Cohn JS. Triglycerides: A risk factor for coronary heart disease. *Atherosclerosis* 1996;124(suppl):S57–S64.

Ebenbichler CF, Kirchmair R, Egger C, et al. Postprandial state and atherosclerosis. *Curr Opin Lipidol* 1995;6:286–290.

Franceschini G, Paoletti R. Pharmacological control of hypertriglyceridemia. *Cardiovasc Drugs Ther* 1993;7:297–302.

Hamsten A, Karpe F. Triglycerides and coronary heart disease—has epidemiology given us the right answer? In: Betteridge DJ, ed. *Lipids: Current Perspectives*. St. Louis: Mosby, 1996:43–68.

Havel RJ. Plasma triglycerides and the clinician: Time for reassessment. *J Am Coll Cardiol* 1998;31:1258–1259.

Kesäniemi YA. Serum triglycerides and clinical benefit in lipid-lowering trials. *Am J Cardiol* 1998;81(4A):70B–73B.

Krauss RM. Atherogenicity of triglyceride-rich lipoproteins. *Am J Cardiol* 1998;81(suppl 4A):13B–17B.

Patsch W, Gotto AM Jr. High-density lipoprotein cholesterol, plasma triglyceride, and coronary heart disease: Pathophysiology and management. *Adv Pharmacol* 1995;32:375–427.

1.8.6 Lipid-Regulating Trials

Blankenhorn DH, Hodis HN. Arterial imaging and atherosclerosis reversal. George Lyman Duff Memorial Lecture. *Arterioscler Thromb* 1994;14:177–192.

Buchwald H, Matts JP, Fitch LL, et al., for the Program on the Surgical Control of the Hyperlipidemias (POSCH) Group. Changes in sequential coronary arteriograms and subsequent coronary events. *JAMA* 1992;268:1429–1433.

Carmena R. [Regression of coronary atherosclerosis: does it exist?] *Rev Esp Cardiol* 1994;47:505–508.

Criqui MH. Triglycerides and cardiovascular disease: A focus on clinical trials. *Eur Heart J* 1998;19(suppl A):A36–A39.

Delanty N, Vaughan CJ. Vascular effects of statins in stroke. *Stroke* 1997;28:2315–2320.

Denke MA. Cholesterol-lowering diets: A review of the evidence. *Arch Intern Med* 1995;155:17–26.

Downs JR, Clearfield M, Weis S, et al. Primary prevention of acute coronary events with lovastatin in men and women with average cholesterol levels. Results of AFCAPS/TexCAPS. *JAMA* 1998;279:1615–1622.

Frick MH, Elo O, Haapa K, et al. Helsinki Heart Study: Primary-prevention trial with gemfibrozil in middle-aged men with dyslipidemia. Safety of treatment, changes in risk factors, and incidence of coronary heart disease. *N Engl J Med* 1987;317:1237–1245.

Lipid Research Clinics Program. The Lipid Research Clinics Coronary Primary Prevention Trial results. I. Reduction in incidence of coronary heart disease. *JAMA* 1984;251:351–364.

Lipid Research Clinics Program. The Lipid Research Clinics Coronary Primary Prevention Trial results. II. The relationship of reduction in incidence of coronary heart disease to cholesterol lowering. *JAMA* 1984;251:365–374.

The Long-Term Intervention with Pravastatin in Ischaemic Disease (LIPID) Study Group. Prevention of cardiovascular events and death with pravastatin in patients with coronary heart disease and a broad range of initial cholesterol levels. *N Engl J Med* 1998;339:1349–1357.

Pitt B, Waters D, Brown WV, et al. Aggressive lipid-lowering therapy compared with angioplasty in stable coronary artery disease. *N Engl J Med* 1999;341:70–76.

Plehn JF, Davis BR, Sacks FM, et al. Reduction of stroke incidence after myocardial infarction with pravastatin. The Cholesterol and Recurrent Events (CARE) study. *Circulation* 1999;99:216–223.

Riegger G, Abletshauser C, Ludwig M, et al. The effect of fluvastatin on cardiac events in patients with symptomatic coronary artery disease during one year of treatment. *Atherosclerosis* 1999;144:263–270.

Rifkind BM. Clinical trials of reducing low-density lipoprotein concentrations. *Endocrinol Metab Clin North Am* 1998;27:585–595.

Rubins HB, Robins SJ, Collins D, et al., for the Veterans Affairs High-Density Lipoprotein Cholesterol Intervention Trial Study Group. Gemfibrozil for the secondary prevention of coronary heart disease in men with low levels of high-density lipoprotein cholesterol. *N Engl J Med* 1999;341:410–418.

Sacks FM. Dietary factors. In: Hennekens CH, ed. *Clinical Trials in Cardiovascular Disease.* Philadelphia: W.B. Saunders, 1999:423–431.

Sacks FM, Pfeffer MA, Moye LA, et al. The effect of pravastatin on coronary events after myocardial infarction in patients with average cholesterol levels. *N Engl J Med* 1996;335:1001–1009.

Scandinavian Simvastatin Survival Study Group. Randomised trial of cholesterol lowering in 4444 patients with coronary heart disease: The Scandinavian Simvastatin Survival Study (4S). *Lancet* 1994;344:1383–1389.

Schaefer EJ, Brousseau ME. Diet, lipoproteins, and coronary heart disease. *Endocrinol Metab Clin North Am* 1998;27:711–732.

Shepherd J, Cobbe SM, Ford I, et al., for the West of Scotland Coronary Prevention Study Group. Prevention of coronary heart disease with pravastatin in men with hypercholesterolemia. *N Engl J Med* 1995;333:1301–1307.

Vogel RA. Coronary risk factors, endothelial function, and atherosclerosis: A review. *Clin Cardiol* 1997;20:426–432.

CLINICAL **G**UIDE

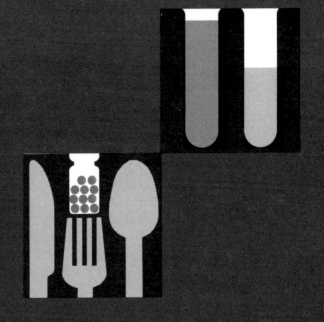

2 Clinical Guide

In recent years, new clinical recommendations for the assessment and management of lipid risk for CHD have been developed by national and international groups of experts to keep pace with a rapidly expanding knowledge base. Key among these documents are the guidelines of the European Atherosclerosis Society and of the U.S. National Cholesterol Education Program. Recommendations for the comprehensive management of multiple lipid and nonlipid risk factors are available from the International Task Force for the Prevention of Coronary Heart Disease/International Atherosclerosis Society (*Nutr Metab Cardiovasc Dis* 1998;8:205–271 or www.chd-taskforce.com) and the Second Joint Task Force of European and Other Societies on Coronary Prevention (*Eur Heart J* 1998;19:1434–1503). Although the objectives and the formulation of these documents are necessarily distinct, there is remarkable agreement among them. These commonalities include an emphasis on the interaction of multiple influences in producing high risk for CHD, and an emphasis on the full implementation of appropriate lifestyle changes as the foundation of therapy.

This Clinical Guide has been developed by the International Lipid Information Bureau to illustrate—in a condensed format—the application of these general principles. It presents the opinion of the ILIB on the step-by-step evaluation and treatment of dyslipidemia, and provides practical guidance on issues that receive differing treatment in the various guidelines. While primarily a synthesis of recently published documents, the Clinical Guide represents the position of the ILIB exclusively.

Many lipid and nonlipid factors stand in continuous relation to CHD risk. The reader should remember that target values or action limits are somewhat arbitrary, and should help patients understand that higher risk does not suddenly begin or end at one value.

Clinical Guide: Stepwise Approach to the Evaluation and Treatment of Dyslipidemia in Adults

	Evaluation and Treatment Steps	Page	For additional information, see Appendixes
2.1	Screen for dyslipidemia	40	C.1, C.2
2.2	Identify and characterize dyslipidemia	42	C.1, C.2
	2.2.1. Concentrations	42	
	2.2.2. Fredrickson phenotyping	44	
2.3	Perform full clinical evaluation	46	C.3
2.4	Estimate the level of overall CHD risk	48	B.1, B.3, B.4
2.5	Treat any underlying conditions and replace or reduce any drugs that can cause secondary dyslipidemia	52	C.2
2.6	Determine any primary dyslipidemia	54	C.2
2.7	Determine the need for dietary intervention and other lifestyle measures	58	D.2–D.5
2.8	Instruct the patient in the cholesterol-lowering diet and risk factor reduction	60	D.1–D.5, D.8
2.9	Consider and select lipid-regulating drug therapy as necessary	64	D.6
	2.9.1. Initiation of therapy	64	
	2.9.2. Selection of agents	67	
2.10	Monitor lipid-regulating interventions	69	D.8

SUMMARY CHARTS
Chart 2-1. Primary Prevention in Adults 70
Chart 2-2. Secondary Prevention in Adults 71

Note: For evaluation and treatment of dyslipidemia in patients with diabetes mellitus and pediatric patients, see Appendixes B.1 and B.2. For special considerations in women and the elderly, see Appendixes B.3 and B.4.

2.1 Screen for Dyslipidemia

Plasma TC should be measured in all adults ($\geq$20 years of age) at least once every 5 years in a selective or opportunistic screening (e.g., on the occasion of a physical examination). The ILIB recommends measurement of HDL-C and TG at the same time, assuming accuracy is ensured. Elevated plasma cholesterol, specifically LDL-C, is one of the strongest risk factors for CHD, and even one measurement of TC is predictive of CHD in epidemiologic studies. The combination of elevated TC or LDL-C and low HDL-C, especially with elevated TG, may confer particularly high risk. LDL-C is calculated using the Friedewald formula (see Table C.1-2 in the Appendixes) if TG is <400 mg/dL (<4.5 mmol/L). If the patient presents in the nonfasting state, TC and HDL-C measurements may still be performed (see Table C.1-1).

Full fasting lipoprotein analysis should always be the first lipid assessment in patients known to have atherosclerotic disease or diabetes mellitus or who are otherwise at high risk for CHD. Evaluation of lipid concentrations should be performed at least annually in patients at high risk. The presence of atherosclerotic disease may be defined as described by the ATP II:

CHD: Definite clinical and laboratory evidence of MI; clinically significant myocardial ischemia; history of coronary artery surgery or coronary angioplasty; or angiogram demonstrating significant coronary atherosclerosis in the presence of clinical symptoms of CHD, although it is not recommended that angiography be performed specifically to classify patients for cholesterol-lowering therapy

PVD: Abdominal aortic aneurysm or clinical signs and symptoms of ischemia of the extremities, accompanied by significant atherosclerosis on angiography or abnormalities of segment-to-arm pressure ratios or flow velocities

Carotid: Cerebral symptoms (TIAs or stroke) accompanied by ultrasound or angiographic demonstration of significant atherosclerosis

Lipid retesting should be performed at regular intervals defined by overall risk. Patients at high risk should be reevaluated in 3–12 months depending on level of risk. Patients without other risk factors with TC <200 mg/dL (<5.2 mmol/L) should be reevaluated within 5 years.

The algorithmic approaches recommended by the ILIB for the assessment and management of dyslipidemia in adults with and without atherosclerotic disease are shown in the summary charts at the end of the Clinical Guide.

2.2 Identify and Characterize Dyslipidemia

2.2.1 Concentrations

Lipid cutpoints are not absolute; they are no more than general advice for risk evaluation and therapy. Many risk factors are continuous variables and interact with one another. Both the number and severity of risk factors should be taken into account in assessing the level of risk. Therapeutic decisions should always be based on the patient's overall risk profile.

As a general rule in observational studies, a 1% decrease in TC yields at least a 2–3% reduction in CHD risk. In primary prevention, TC >200 mg/dL (>5.2 mmol/L) or LDL-C >130 mg/dL (>3.4 mmol/L) generally requires some degree of management. CHD risk is about 2 times higher when TC reaches 240 or 250 mg/dL (6.2 or 6.5 mmol/L) compared with TC of 190 mg/dL (5.0 mmol/L). Hypercholesterolemia is severe when TC reaches about 300 mg/dL (7.8 mmol/L); CHD risk is at least 4 times as high with TC of 300 mg/dL (7.8 mmol/L) compared with TC of 190 mg/dL (5.0 mmol/L). The ATP II has set a lower cutpoint for LDL-C in patients with atherosclerotic disease: LDL-C >100 mg/dL (>2.6 mmol/L) is considered higher than optimal and requires intervention. The Second Joint Task Force uses an LDL-C target of <115 mg/dL (<3.0 mmol/L) for both primary and secondary prevention (see Table A.2-1). On the basis of available clinical data, the ILIB supports an aggressive LDL-C goal in secondary prevention.

HDL-C concentrations are generally higher in women, especially premenopausal women, compared with men. The ATP II provides a general estimate of risk for both sexes at HDL-C <35 mg/dL (<0.9 mmol/L), the Second Joint Task Force at <40 mg/dL (<1.0 mmol/L). The ILIB supports the higher cutpoint. As with TC or LDL-C, the relation between HDL-C and CHD risk is continuously graded over a wide range of values. As a rule of thumb, an increase of 1 mg/dL (0.03 mmol/L) in HDL-C is associated with a 2–3% reduction in CHD risk. It is reinforced by the ILIB that the TC:HDL-C and LDL-C:HDL-C ratios provide useful estimates of risk.

The ILIB considers TG <150 mg/dL (<1.7 mmol/L) to be desirable; higher TG may be associated with increased risk for CHD, particularly when insulin resistance or diabetes is present and HDL-C is low. TG concentrations >1,000 mg/dL (>11.3 mmol/L) confer high risk for acute pancreatitis.

Table 2.2-1. General Cutpoints for Dyslipidemia

Lipid Determination	Primary Prevention		Secondary Prevention	
	Desirable	Needs Attention	Desirable	Needs Attention
Total cholesterol	<200 (<5.2)	>200 (>5.2) Moderately elevated >240 (>6.2) Elevated >300 (>7.8) Severely elevated	(LDL-C should always be determined in patients known to have atherosclerotic disease.)	
LDL-C	<130 (<3.4)	>130 (>3.4) Moderately elevated >160 (>4.1) Elevated >190 (>4.9) Severely elevated	<100 (<2.6)	>100 (>2.6) Elevated
HDL-C	>45 (>1.2)	<40 (<1.0) Low	>45 (>1.2)	<40 (<1.0) Low
TC:HDL-C ratio	<4.5	>5 High	<3.5	>4 High
LDL-C:HDL-C ratio	<3	>3.5 High	<2.5	>3 High
Triglyceride	<150 (<1.7)	>200 (>2.3) Elevated >1,000 (>11.3) Severely elevated (confers risk for acute pancreatitis)	<150 (<1.7)	>200 (>2.3) Elevated >1,000 (>11.3) Severely elevated (confers risk for acute pancreatitis)

Note: All lipid values are mg/dL (mmol/L).

Note: For lipid cutpoints in adults with diabetes mellitus, see Chart B.1-1 and Tables B.1-4 and B.1-5 in the Appendixes.

2.2.2 Fredrickson Phenotyping

The Fredrickson classification of hyperlipidemias is based on the plasma lipoprotein patterns associated with elevated concentrations of cholesterol and/or TG and disregards HDL-C concentration. It relies on separation of lipoproteins by electrophoresis and/or ultracentrifugation combined with precipitation. The major plasma lipoproteins in order of decreasing size and increasing density are chylomicrons, VLDL, IDL, LDL, and HDL (see Table E.1-1 in the Appendixes). The Fredrickson classification is not an etiologic classification of disease and does not differentiate primary and secondary hyperlipidemias, but it has been useful in characterizing lipoprotein abnormalities. The Fredrickson classification distinguishes whether TG elevation represents TG from dietary sources (TG packaged in chylomicrons) or TG-rich particles of endogenous origin (VLDL produced by the liver—for example, in individuals on a high-carbohydrate diet). It is also helpful in the diagnosis of familial type III hyperlipidemia (familial dysbetalipoproteinemia; broad-beta band on lipoprotein electrophoresis) when apo E isoform determination is not available. Establishing the lipoprotein phenotype present does not substitute for making a diagnosis of the underlying cause. That studies are still carried out using the Fredrickson classification indicates a focus on the abnormal lipoprotein profile rather than a specific disease etiology.

Table 2.2-2. Fredrickson Classification of the Hyperlipidemias

Phenotype	Lipoprotein(s) Elevated	Plasma Cholesterol Concentration	Plasma TG Concentration	Atherogenicity	Relative Frequency*
I	Chylomicrons	Normal to ↑	↑↑↑	Rarely seen	<1%
IIa	LDL	↑↑	Normal	+++	10%
IIb	LDL and VLDL	↑↑	↑↑	+++	40%
III	IDL	↑↑	↑↑↑	+++	<1%
IV	VLDL	Normal to ↑	↑↑	+	45%
V	VLDL and chylomicrons	↑ to ↑↑	↑↑↑↑	+	5%

*Approximate percentages of U.S. patients with hyperlipidemia.

2.3 Perform Full Clinical Evaluation

Full clinical evaluation should be performed in patients without athero-sclerotic disease when: 1) LDL-C exceeds 130 mg/dL (3.4 mmol/L) and other risk is present; 2) LDL-C exceeds 160 mg/dL (4.1 mmol/L) regardless of other risk; 3) the LDL-C:HDL-C ratio exceeds 3.5; or 4) TG exceeds 200 mg/dL (2.3 mmol/L) and other risk is present (see Chart 2-1, page 70). In patients with atherosclerotic disease, full clinical evaluation should be undertaken when 1) LDL-C exceeds 100 mg/dL (2.6 mmol/L), 2) HDL-C is below 40 mg/dL (1.0 mmol/L), or 3) TG exceeds 200 mg/dL (2.3 mmol/L) (see Chart 2-2, page 71).

The aim of the clinical evaluation is to gather sufficient information to select therapy properly. This includes attempting to determine the root cause or causes of the dyslipidemia, whether the dyslipidemia is primary or secondary. A more complete evaluation of risk factor and cardiovascular status should be made at this time. Major CHD risk factors in addition to hyperlipidemia are listed in Table 2.4-1. Also noted should be conditions unrelated to CHD risk that might influence selection of therapy, including competing illnesses or conditions that might be deleteriously affected by therapy. Concurrent medications should be taken into account. Obtaining a comprehensive profile can help anticipate potential difficulties and thereby facilitate institution of therapy. Causes of secondary dyslipidemia (see 2.5) must be excluded in this process, especially hypothyroidism, diabetes mellitus, excessive alcohol intake, renal abnormalities, and obstructive liver disease.

Table 2.3-1. Clinical Evaluation

Component	Notes
Establish personal history	Including CVD, hypertension, and dyslipidemia. Patients with atherosclerotic disease or type 2 diabetes mellitus are at highest risk for CHD events.
Take family history, and always consider familial dyslipidemias	Determine family history of CVD, dyslipidemia, hypertension, diabetes mellitus, central obesity; see Table C.3-1 in the Appendixes for step-by-step family history. Family testing is essential to the diagnosis of familial disorders; see 2.6 for selected primary dyslipidemias.
Evaluate diet and other lifestyle components	Daily total energy intake and intake of total fat, saturated fat and other types of fat, cholesterol, alcohol, simple carbohydrates, and sodium; type and amount of physical exercise; smoking habits; stress
Perform physical examination	Including weight, height, calculated BMI (weight/height^2 in kg/m^2; normal weight, 18.5–24.9 kg/m^2), waist:hip ratio (desirable <0.9 men, <0.8 women) or even simple waist circumference ($\geq$94 cm in men, $\geq$80 cm in women), blood pressure, examination for manifestations of atherosclerosis (e.g., vascular bruits, reduced peripheral pulses), manifestations of dyslipidemia (e.g., corneal arcus, xanthelasmas/xanthomas, hepatosplenomegaly), and thyroid abnormalities
Perform laboratory and other tests	Full fasting lipoprotein analysis (TC, HDL-C, TG, calculated LDL-C) and routine laboratory evaluations, among them creatine kinase, fasting blood glucose, alkaline phosphatase, liver function and thyroid tests, urinalysis, and ECG
Establish risk factor profile	High risk is often due to multiple risk factors, less often due to a single risk factor severe in degree; consider age and gender. See 2.4 for major risk factors, as well as Appendix C.2 regarding common causes and presentations of hyperlipidemia.

2.4 Estimate the Level of Overall CHD Risk

It bears repeating that while treatment algorithms delineate broad categories of risk, several variables (lipids, lipoproteins, blood pressure, BMI, and age) associated with CHD risk are continuous. Clinical judgment is required for risk assessment in any given individual. The presence of multiple risk factors is of particular concern and should be weighted appropriately when considering follow-up. Multiple risk factors tend to increase risk in a synergistic rather than an additive manner. Risk calculators may be useful but do not replace complete clinical evaluation and clinical judgment.

Major CHD risk factors that must be considered in the clinical evaluation in addition to hyperlipidemia are listed on the next page. A number of other factors have been associated with the development of CHD, notably elevated plasma **fibrinogen** (an independent CHD risk factor that may contribute to a hypercoagulable state and that can result from smoking), elevated plasma **Lp[a]**, elevated plasma **homocysteine**, and, in subjects with diabetes mellitus or insulin resistance, **microalbuminuria**. In the individual, elevation of fibrinogen (the measurement of which is not always reliable) must be interpreted with caution because transient elevation is common in intercurrent acute illness as part of the acute phase response. There is evidence that the presence of small, dense LDL associated with high plasma apo B could markedly increase CHD risk. Among other possible risk factors are physical inactivity, heavy ethanol consumption, hyperglycemia, fasting hyperinsulinemia, insulin resistance, social and psychologic factors such as hostility and stressful life events, and other thrombogenic factors such as von Willebrand factor, factor VII, and plasminogen activator inhibitor 1 (PAI-1). Some of these have not been clearly shown to be independent risk factors, and for some, measurements are not yet widely performed or useful. The clinician may wish to consider them, however, in estimating overall CHD risk in the patient. In premenopausal women, use of oral contraceptives is associated with increased risk for CVD in smokers, particularly in women older than 35.

Table 2.4-1. Major CHD Risk Factors That Must Be Considered in Addition to Hyperlipidemia in the Clinical Evaluation

Age (≥45 in men, postmenopausal status in women)

Personal history of CVD

Cigarette smoking

Hypertension

Diabetes mellitus

Family history of premature CHD

Low HDL-C: <40 mg/dL (<1.0 mmol/L)

Abdominal obesity

Table 2.4-2. Assessment of Patient's Overall Risk for CHD

Clinical Judgment*	Quantitative Risk Estimate According to PROCAM Algorithm†	
	Risk Quintile (Figure 2.4-1)	Approx. Annual Absolute Risk in Middle-aged Men
Small increase in risk		
• Presence of 1 major risk factor of moderate degree in patient without known atherosclerotic disease *(example: middle-aged man with TC 200–300 mg/dL [5.2–7.8 mmol/L] with no nonlipid risk factors, or TC:HDL-C 4.5–5, or smoking about 10 cigarettes/day with no other risk factors)*	3rd	0.3%
Moderate increase in risk		
• Presence of 1 major risk factor of severe degree in patient without known atherosclerotic disease *(example: middle-aged man smoking about 20 cigarettes/ day)*, OR • Presence of 2 major risk factors of moderate degree in patient without known atherosclerotic disease *(example: middle-aged man with TC 200–300 mg/dL [5.2–7.8 mmol/L] plus HDL-C <40 mg/dL [<1.0 mmol/L] or plus obesity)*	4th	0.7%
High risk		
• Presence of atherosclerotic disease, OR in patient without known atherosclerotic disease: • Presence of type 2 diabetes mellitus, OR • Presence of a major genetic lipid disorder associated with premature atherosclerotic disease, OR • Presence of 2 major risk factors of severe degree, OR • Presence of ≥3 major risk factors of moderate degree	5th	2.3%

Source: Data modified from The International Task Force for Prevention of Coronary Heart Disease. Coronary heart disease: Reducing the risk. The scientific background for primary and secondary prevention of coronary heart disease. A worldwide view. *Nutr Metab Cardiovasc Dis* 1998;8:205–271.

Note: The goal of risk assessment is to assign an appropriate type and intensity of treatment of a risk factor. In the case of lipid risk factors, this implies decisions as to how vigorous a diet is needed, whether a drug is required and if so at what dosage, and what target values to aim for. This may be achieved by judging whether the patient is at average risk or whether she or he falls into one of the above grades of increased risk. Risk factors are judged by both number and severity. The greater the risk for CHD, the lower the target value for LDL-C, and the more vigorous the treatment required.

*Other risk correlates such as elevated plasma fibrinogen (see 2.4) may be considered in addition to major risk factors.

†Risk calculator for use in primary prevention, based on 8-year data from the prospective, observational epidemiologic Münster Heart Study (PROCAM), available at www.chd-taskforce.com; risk factors included are age, LDL-C, HDL-C, fasting TG, SBP, and presence or absence of cigarette smoking, diabetes mellitus, and family history of MI. Another recent risk algorithm for use in primary prevention is based on Framingham Study data (Wilson et al. *Circulation* 1998;97:1837–1847 or www.nhlbi.nih.gov/about/framingham/riskabs.htm). Use of mathematical risk calculators may supplement but does not replace clinical judgment. (See also Table 3-1, page 103.)

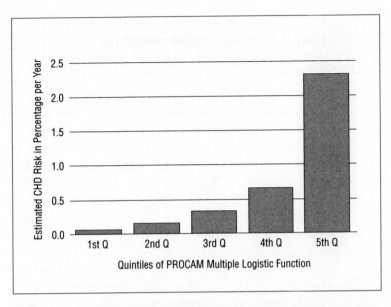

Figure 2.4-1. Estimated risk for a CHD event (fatal or nonfatal MI or sudden cardiac death), expressed as quintiles of multiple logistic function, among men aged 40–65 years in the Münster Heart Study (PROCAM). There were 248 coronary events in 8 years among 4,639 men recruited from 1979 to 1985. Risk between quintile 1 and quintile 5 differs by 40-fold. From the International Task Force for Prevention of Coronary Heart Disease. Coronary heart disease: Reducing the risk. The scientific background for primary and secondary prevention of coronary heart disease. A worldwide view. *Nutr Metab Cardiovasc Dis* 1998;8:205–271 (also available at www.chd-taskforce.com); used with permission.

2.5 Treat Any Underlying Conditions and Replace or Reduce Any Drugs That Can Cause Secondary Dyslipidemia

In addition to lifestyle factors, common causes of secondary dyslipidemia include diabetes mellitus, nephrotic syndrome, chronic renal failure, and hypothyroidism, as well as some drug treatments. Protease inhibitor administration may cause large increases in TG and LDL-C, and may be associated with glucose intolerance, diabetes mellitus, and lipodystrophy.

Most dyslipidemias are of polygenic, multifactorial origin. If dyslipidemia persists despite treatment of causes of secondary dyslipidemia, treat as a primary lipid disorder.

Decreased HDL-C may be related to HTG, obesity, a sedentary lifestyle, cigarette smoking, or impaired glucose tolerance. Although the HTG–low HDL-C syndrome is frequent, it usually requires specialized diagnostics to unravel whether the hypoalphalipoproteinemia is primary or secondary in origin. Drugs that can decrease HDL-C (most also increasing TG) include acne medications (vitamin A derivatives, e.g., isotretinoin), anabolic steroids, progestins, testosterone, and beta-blockers without intrinsic sympathomimetic activity. Causes of secondary hyperalphalipoproteinemia include cholesteryl ester transfer protein (CETP) deficiency, the use of antiepileptic medications, and pesticide exposure.

Addressing lifestyle factors is discussed in 2.7 and 2.8, as well as in related Appendixes.

Table 2.5-1. Selected Causes of Secondary Hyperlipidemia

Related to Plasma Cholesterol Elevation

    Diet rich in saturated fatty acids
    Hypothyroidism
    Nephrotic syndrome
    Chronic liver disease (mainly primary biliary cirrhosis)
    Cholestasis
    Monoclonal gammopathy
    Cushing's syndrome
    Oral contraceptive use
    Anorexia nervosa
    Acute intermittent porphyria
    Protease inhibitor use

Related to Plasma Triglyceride Elevation

    Diet rich in carbohydrates
    Excessive alcohol consumption
    Obesity
    Pregnancy
    Diabetes mellitus
    Hypothyroidism
    Chronic renal failure
    Pancreatitis
    Bulimia
    Cushing's syndrome
    Hypopituitarism
    Monoclonal gammopathy
    Glycogen storage disease
    Lipodystrophy
    Acute intermittent porphyria
    Systemic lupus erythematosus
    Beta-blocker, diuretic use (see Table D.6-8)
    Estrogen use (contraceptive or replacement)
    Glucocorticoid use
    Isotretinoin use
    Protease inhibitor use
    Tamoxifen use

2.6 Determine Any Primary Dyslipidemia

The genetic lipid disorders most often identified in clinical practice are FCH, polygenic hypercholesterolemia, FH, and type III hyperlipidemia. Examination for manifestations of dyslipidemia (e.g., corneal arcus, xanthelasmas/xanthomas, hepatosplenomegaly) as well as for manifestations of atherosclerosis (e.g., vascular bruits, reduced peripheral pulses) is always important.

Searching for a genetic origin through specialized laboratory methods can be useful in family counseling. Dyslipidemias are most often polygenic and multifactorial in origin. Various genetic abnormalities, some of which can be identified in specialized laboratories, impart a genetic predisposition to dyslipidemia and atherosclerosis. If dyslipidemia occurs in young adults, efforts should be undertaken to identify the possible genetic origins of disease, which often becomes manifest only in the presence of exogenous or environmental factors. Homozygous FH is manifested early in life and may be detected at birth. Heterozygous FH merits particular attention because it is a frequent and potentially lethal disorder associated with premature atherosclerosis (third and fourth decades). It may have increased frequency in certain populations because of the presence of a founder effect.

Table 2.6-1. Selected Primary Dyslipidemias

Disorder*	Fredrickson Phenotype(s)	Transmission and Mechanism	Estimated Prevalence	Major Clinical Findings	Treatment Principles
Familial chylomicronemia	I	Autosomal recessive; lipoprotein lipase or apo C-II deficiency	Rare	Usually diagnosed in childhood by recurrent abdominal pain and pancreatitis. Lipemia retinalis, eruptive xanthomas, hepatosplenomegaly, and occasionally peripheral neuropathy and reversible mental changes may occur. Heterozygotes: Normal TG or mild HTG in absence of other conditions associated with HTG. Homozygotes: Fasting TG may exceed 1,000 mg/dL (11.3 mmol/L). Has only rarely been linked to increased CHD risk.	Diet low in simple carbohydrates and fat (<10% of total energy intake as fat); avoidance of alcohol; weight control; intake of medium-chain TG helpful; drug therapy usually not helpful
Heterozygous familial hypercholesterolemia (FH)	IIa (IIb rare)	Autosomal dominant; LDL receptor defect	1/500	TC elevated at birth, eventually reaches 350–500 mg/dL (9.0–12.9 mmol/L). Tendon xanthomas, corneal arcus, and premature atherosclerosis are typical.	Diet plus drug therapy (usually a statin alone or statin plus resin); LDL apheresis in severe cases
Homozygous familial hypercholesterolemia (FH)	IIa (IIb rare)	Autosomal dominant; LDL receptor defect	$1/10^6$	TC elevated at birth; TC reaches 700–1,200 mg/dL (18.1–31.0 mmol/L); cutaneous xanthomas, tendon xanthomas; corneal arcus; severe, widespread early atherosclerosis, including aortic stenosis.	Resistant to diet and most drug therapy; atorvastatin may be used singly or in combination with LDL apheresis. Additional therapies such as LDL apheresis, liver transplantation

Continued on next page

*All hyperlipidemias except familial chylomicronemia are typically associated with increased risk for CHD (variable in familial HTG); see Table 2.2-2.

Table 2.6-1. Selected Primary Dyslipidemias—Continued

Disorder*	Fredrickson Phenotype(s)	Transmission and Mechanism	Estimated Prevalence	Major Clinical Findings	Treatment Principles
Familial defective apo B-100	IIa	Autosomal dominant; apo B mutation	Prevalence varies by ethnicity; rare to 1/600	Lipoprotein values and clinical features can resemble heterozygous FH; in some cases, may be more moderate; definitive diagnosis by molecular analysis.	Treat as in heterozygous FH; diet plus statin and/or resin
Polygenic hypercholesterolemia	IIa	Mode of transmission unknown; various genetic defects	High, but depends on definition	TC elevation generally less than in heterozygous FH; when elevated HDL-C ruled out, as many as 80% of patients with isolated hypercholesterolemia have polygenic hypercholesterolemia.	Dependent on LDL-C value, sex, age, and CHD status. Severe cases treated as in heterozygous FH (combination-drug therapy may not be necessary)
Familial combined hyperlipidemia (FCH)	IIa, IIb, IV	Heterogeneous disease of still unknown etiology; associated with overproduction of apo B in most cases and with plasma hyperapobetalipoproteinemia (hyper–apo B)	Approx.1/100	Elevated TC or TG (or both) in patient and family members. When TC elevated, typically 250–350 mg/dL (6.5–9.1 mmol/L); when TG elevated, 2/3 of patients have mild to moderate HTG, but elevation may be severe; no unique clinical features; may or may not be expressed in childhood.	Follow standard clinical guidelines for hypercholesterolemia, HTG, or combined hyperlipidemia

Disorder	Type	Genetics/Mechanism	Frequency	Clinical and Laboratory Features	Management
Type III hyperlipidemia (familial dysbetalipoproteinemia†)	III	Usually mimics autosomal recessive mode; an apo E-linked metabolic defect (E2/2 phenotype), usually requiring other metabolic factors for full expression (1% of the general population is homozygous for E2)	1/5,000	Typically, TC 300–600 mg/dL (7.8–15.5 mmol/L), TG 400–800 mg/dL (4.5–9.0 mmol/L) (TG may be much higher); palmar xanthomas, tuberoeruptive xanthomas may occur; disorder is exacerbated by diabetes mellitus, other disorders; not commonly expressed in childhood; specialized laboratory can provide definitive diagnosis (apo E isoform); premature CHD, PVD, and stroke.	Diet low in saturated fat, weight control; drug therapy to reduce remnant lipoproteins—fibrates are first-choice drugs; niacin may be considered if diabetes mellitus or prediabetic condition is absent
Familial endogenous hypertriglyceridemia (FHTG; type IV hyperlipidemia) and familial mixed hypertriglyceridemia (type V hyperlipidemia)	IV, V	Often dominant; mechanism not established	Phenotype IV Approx.1/300; phenotype V rare	Typically, TG 200–500 mg/dL (2.3–5.6 mmol/L) in phenotype IV, TG >1,000 mg/dL (>11.3 mmol/L) in phenotype V; uncommonly, "pure" type IV (no chylomicrons) with TG >1,000 mg/dL (>11.3 mmol/L), HDL-C usually decreased; early CHD in some families but not in others. FHTG (type IV hyperlipidemia) is often associated with a modest chylomicronemia, giving a type V pattern in which the VLDL fraction remains predominant; to be distinguished from severe chylomicronemia associated with elevated VLDL (type V hyperlipidemia), a separate entity although probably heterogeneous in origin.	Follow standard clinical guidelines for HTG
Familial low HDL-C (hypoalphalipoproteinemia)‡		Usually dominant; molecular basis elucidated for some, but etiology unclear in others	Very rare	"Familial low HDL-C" is an interim term; marked differences in association with premature CHD. Clinical differences include HDL deficiencies with corneal opacities; xanthomatosis; tonsil anomalies, neuropathy, and hepatosplenomegaly; amyloidosis.	Heterogeneous group; refer to lipid specialist

*All hyperlipidemias except familial chylomicronemia are typically associated with increased risk for CHD (variable in familial HTG); see Table 2.2-2.
†Dysbetalipoproteinemia indicates the presence of remnants of chylomicrons and VLDL.
‡Only some of the familial low HDL-C syndromes described thus far by investigators have been associated with increased risk for atherosclerosis.

2.7 Determine the Need for Dietary Intervention and Other Lifestyle Measures

Instruct **all** patients in risk factor reduction and prevention, including improved eating patterns with reduction of saturated fat, *trans* fatty acids, and dietary cholesterol, weight loss in the overweight or prevention of overweight, increased physical activity as appropriate, and cessation or prevention of smoking. The general cholesterol-lowering diet (Table 2.8-1) is recommended for the general population age 2 years and older. Patients with atherosclerotic disease should begin dietary intervention with intensified diet. Implementation of a heart-healthy diet is discussed in Appendix D.2. Weight control, physical activity, and smoking cessation are discussed in Appendixes D.3, D.4, and D.5.

Table 2.7-1. Lipid Goals for Lifestyle Intervention

Lipid Determination	Primary Prevention	Secondary Prevention
Total cholesterol	<200 (<5.2)	
LDL-C	<130 (<3.4)	<100 (<2.6)
HDL-C	>45 (>1.2)	>45 (>1.2)
TC:HDL-C ratio	<4.5	<3.5
LDL-C:HDL-C ratio	<3	<2.5
Triglyceride*	<150 (<1.7)	<150 (<1.7)

Note: All lipid values are mg/dL (mmol/L).
Note: On the basis of current evidence, the ILIB believes that low HDL-C and elevated TG should each be targeted for therapy.
Note: For lipid goals in adults with diabetes mellitus, see Tables B.1-4 and B.1-5.
*When TG exceeds 1,000 (11.3), the TG goal is <200 (<2.3) but that goal is not easily achieved in these patients.

2.8 Instruct the Patient in the Cholesterol-Lowering Diet and Risk Factor Reduction

Dietary intervention is the cornerstone of therapy for dyslipidemia. Judiciously employed, it is a risk-free measure whose efficacy has been demonstrated in clinical trials. In many patients, lipid disorders can be managed with lifestyle changes, including diet, weight control, regular physical exercise, and smoking cessation. Lifestyle measures are often associated with additional benefits, such as reduced blood pressure and improved glucose tolerance, and they should be emphasized for all patients. Although lifestyle has a strong influence on CHD rates, dyslipidemia with a strong genetic component is frequently not normalized by lifestyle changes.

The general cholesterol-lowering diet shown here and the NCEP Step I Diet (see Table A.1-7) are essentially identical. These guidelines were developed to apply to populations consuming a western or westernized diet; for other cultures, they may need considerable adaptation. The key elements are decreases in saturated fat and dietary cholesterol. When the general cholesterol-lowering diet is initiated in patients consuming a typical western diet, on average a 10% decrease in LDL-C may be expected. Not infrequently, however, major decreases in LDL-C can be achieved by diet alone. Response is highly variable: the range of response encompasses both hyporesponders and hyperresponders. With good dietary compliance, plasma cholesterol improvements are seen within about 2 weeks in general, and in some patients almost immediately. Some patients, however, are able to make dietary changes only gradually. Improvement of the general eating pattern should also include reduced sodium intake and avoidance of excess alcohol intake. A heart-healthy eating pattern low in saturated fat is recommended for the general population age 2 years and older as a preventive. Diet may have beneficial cardiovascular consequences beyond its effects on lipid concentrations (e.g., antithrombotic, antioxidant, improved endothelial function). Dietary changes should be pursued even when effects on LDL-C concentrations are minimal.

Patients with atherosclerotic disease should begin dietary intervention with intensified diet (shown, or the NCEP Step II Diet, outlined in Table A.1-7). An intensified diet usually requires involvement of a dietitian or other qualified nutrition expert to ensure compliance and (especially in the elderly) adequate nutrition. At any dietary level, the involvement of a qualified nutrition expert is often helpful. Because dyslipidemia is typically asymptomatic, regular follow-up is necessary to reinforce motivation and ensure compliance.

Table 2.8-1. The Cholesterol-Lowering Diet

Component	Recommended Intake, % of Total Energy* General†	Recommended Intake, % of Total Energy* Intensified‡	Notes
Total fat	≤30%	25–27%	• The World Health Organization recommends that total fat intake not be <15% of energy intake. The American Heart Association endorses that recommendation. • The American Academy of Pediatrics recommends that total fat intake not be <20% in the pediatric population.
SFA	≤10%	6–8%	• SFA intake is the strongest dietary determinant of plasma LDL-C concentration.§ • High content: butterfat (cheese, cream, whole milk, etc.); fat of beef, pork, lamb, poultry; palm, palm kernel, coconut oils
MUFA		10–15%	• Oleic acid, found in olive oil, canola oil, and high-oleic forms of sunflower and safflower seed oils, as well as in avocados and nuts, is the major source of MUFA in the diet. High intake of oleic acid appears to be safe. • Avoid *trans* fatty acids, which raise LDL-C more than the native oils and less than SFA. High content: shortening, some margarines, and foods such as fried foods and cookies prepared with these fats
PUFA		No more than 7–10%	• Omega-6 fatty acids: Data are not available to support safety of increased intake of linoleic acid. High content: soybean oil, corn oil, high-linoleic forms of sunflower and safflower seed oils • Omega-3 fatty acids: Consumption of cold-water fish rich in omega-3 fatty acids is encouraged (e.g., Atlantic herring, Atlantic mackerel, sockeye salmon, whiting, rainbow trout, and albacore tuna).

Calories	Reduce when weight loss needed	• Consumption of excess calories leads to obesity, which is frequently accompanied by increased TG, decreased HDL-C, and the appearance of small, dense LDL. Not all fat-free and low-fat foods are low in calories.
Cholesterol	<300 mg/day	<200–250 mg/day	• Dietary cholesterol definitely raises LDL-C in some individuals. Major sources are egg yolk and meat (lean and fatty). Focus on decrease of egg yolk, animal fat, and organ meat.
Carbohydrate	Approx. 55%	• In large amounts, CHO (vs. MUFA) raises TG and reduces HDL-C. Avoid excessive sugar. Diets high in refined CHO are often high in calories and low in complex CHO, fiber, and essential vitamins and minerals. Emphasize consumption of complex CHO in the form of vegetables, grains, and legumes; 25–30 g/day dietary fiber from foods (not supplements) is recommended.
Protein	Approx. 15%	• Select sources of protein that are low in SFA.

Note: CHO = carbohydrate; MUFA = monounsaturated fatty acids; PUFA = polyunsaturated fatty acids; SFA = saturated fatty acids.

Note: For cardiovascular health, it is also advisable to limit sodium and alcohol, especially if high blood pressure is present. Daily sodium intake should be <2,400 mg, lower when renal disease is present. When alcohol is not contraindicated, daily consumption should not exceed 30 mL (24 g, or 1 fl oz) ethanol (~2 drinks) for men, or 15 mL (12 g, or 0.5 fl oz) ethanol (~1 drink) for women and lighter-weight men. Patients with HTG may need more detailed dietary guidance, and HDL-C concentration is generally little affected by changes in dietary fat.

*Calories from alcohol are not included.

†Recommended for the general population age 2 years and older.

‡The intensified diet is initial dietary therapy in secondary prevention, as well as in primary-prevention patients already complying with the general cholesterol-lowering diet.

§According to the Hegsted equation, the change in plasma TC (ΔTC, mg/dL) in response to a change in the composition of the diet is given by ΔTC = 2.16 ΔSFA – 1.65 ΔPUFA + 0.068 Δdietary cholesterol, where SFA and PUFA are the percentages of calories derived from SFA and PUFA and dietary cholesterol is mg/day.

•

2.9 Consider and Select Lipid-Regulating Drug Therapy as Necessary

2.9.1 Initiation of Therapy

Lipid-regulating drug therapy supplements rather than replaces lifestyle changes. The physician needs to consider a variety of factors carefully before beginning drug therapy, including the patient's overall risk for CHD, the potential for adverse effects and drug interactions, and the cost of such therapy, in particular, because lipid-regulating therapy is usually long-term or lifelong. The available pharmacologic options, each offering a favorable risk:benefit ratio, allow drug therapy to be tailored to the specific lipid abnormality of an individual patient. Lipid-regulating drug therapy is underused, and physicians should be more diligent in applying this proven therapy. Clinical judgment is required as well to recognize patients for whom lipid-regulating drug therapy is not appropriate, including patients with limited life expectancy. High-risk but otherwise healthy elderly patients are candidates for lipid-regulating pharmacotherapy.

Four questions to consider before beginning lipid-regulating drug therapy are:

- Is the workup complete?
- Have the lipid goals been determined?
- Has instruction about diet and other lifestyle changes been given?
- Does the agent selected match the lipid disorder and the risk level?

The length of a trial of lifestyle measures alone depends on the overall risk of the patient. For example, the use of lifestyle alone may last >1 year in a young man or premenopausal woman whose LDL-C elevation is not severe and who has no other risk. The higher the CHD risk, the shorter the trial of lifestyle measures alone. Drug therapy may begin at the same time as the institution of lifestyle measures in individuals at high risk. Given the impressive outcomes of recent clinical trials of statins (see Introduction), some authorities believe that withholding statin therapy in an effort to reach target LDL-C with lifestyle changes is not necessary when LDL-C exceeds 130 mg/dL (3.4 mmol/L) in secondary prevention. The addition of drug therapy before hospital release may also be advantageous in terms of compliance. It should be remembered that in an infarct patient, lipid determinations need to be made no later than 24 hours after the event (preferably at admission or within 12 hours; see Table C.1-1 in the Appendixes).

The initiation levels given on the next page are not absolute and should be interpreted in the context of the overall clinical status of the patient. The LDL-C goal should be low in secondary prevention. Several trials of various magnitude (see Introduction) are congruent in supporting the notion that drug therapy to lower plasma TG and/or raise HDL-C is associated with decreased coronary atherosclerosis progression (BECAIT, LOCAT, LCAS) and a reduced CHD event rate (Helsinki Heart Study, AFCAPS/TexCAPS, HIT, BECAIT). In isolated low HDL-C, drug therapy is not generally recommended in primary prevention but may be considered in secondary prevention. There is growing evidence that beneficial cardiovascular effects of lipid-regulating drugs may be mediated by mechanisms other than atherosclerosis regression. These effects, referred to as *pleiotropic effects,* include improvement in endothelial dysfunction, antioxidant effects, and plaque stabilization (see Appendix E.2.4).

Dosages, lipid effects, and side effects of lipid-regulating agents as well as potential interactions are described in Appendix D.6. Cost effectiveness is discussed in D.9. Additional considerations in population subsets appear in Appendixes B.1–B.4, and D.8 provides ways to enhance compliance.

Table 2.9-1. Initiation Levels and Goals for Lipid-Regulating Drug Therapy

Patient Group	Initiation*	Goal	
		Desirable	**Minimal (If Different)**
Primary prevention†			
Other risk absent	LDL-C >190 (>4.9)‡	LDL-C <130 (<3.4)	LDL-C <160 (<4.1)
Other risk present	LDL-C >160 (>4.1)	LDL-C <130 (<3.4)	
Other risk high	TG >200 (>2.3)	TG <150 (<1.7)	TG <200 (<2.3)
Secondary prevention			
All patients	LDL-C >130 (>3.4)	LDL-C <100 (<2.6)	
	TG >200 (>2.3)	TG <150 (<1.7)	TG <200 (<2.3)

Note: All lipid values are mg/dL (mmol/L).

Note: In general, drug therapy is considered only after an adequate trial of lifestyle intervention. However, according to a number of authorities, withholding statin therapy in an effort to reach target LDL-C with lifestyle changes is not necessary for LDL-C >130 (>3.4) in secondary prevention; other authorities still prefer a brief trial of lifestyle changes (4–6 weeks) in these patients. A brief (6-week) trial of lifestyle therapy is recommended when LDL-C is between 100 and 130 (2.6–3.4) in secondary prevention.

Note: HDL-C <40 (<1.0) needs attention. Drug therapy intended solely to raise HDL-C is generally not recommended in primary prevention unless CHD segregates with low HDL-C in the family, but may be considered in secondary prevention. HDL-C concentration is also considered in drug selection and dosage.

Note: At present there is no drug available that is effective in chylomicronemia, a condition in which TG may exceed 1,000 (11.3).

Note: Drug therapy recommendations for adults with diabetes mellitus are provided in Table B.1-6 in the Appendixes.

*The physician must use individualized clinical judgment in patients who do not meet criteria for drug therapy but who have not attained goals with lifestyle changes.

†Also consider drug therapy if the LDL-C:HDL-C ratio remains >3.5–4 despite an adequate trial of lifestyle intervention. See 2.4 regarding estimation of overall risk for CHD.

‡When LDL-C is 190–220 (4.9–5.7) and there is *no other risk,* consider delaying drug therapy in both men <35 years old and premenopausal women.

2.9.2 Selection of Agents

All classes of available lipid-regulating drugs—HMG-CoA reductase inhibitors (statins), bile-acid sequestrants (resins), nicotinic acid (niacin), and fibric-acid derivatives (fibrates)—are clinically safe and effective. In addition to considerations such as cost, availability, side effects, and potential interactions, drug selection depends on the lipid or lipids targeted for intervention, as well as the degree of correction needed.

The statins, resins, and niacin exert the greatest LDL-C-lowering effect; the statins are a breakthrough in the treatment of hypercholesterolemia. The fibrates and niacin are the most effective agents for TG lowering. However, the EAS considers niacin, as a single agent, to be of limited usefulness because of its poor tolerability at adequate dosages; in addition, niacin has a relative contraindication in diabetes mellitus or hyperuricemia. The fibrates and niacin have the most powerful HDL-C-raising effects. The statins have moderate effects in lowering TG and raising HDL-C; the effect on plasma TG concentration is proportional to the baseline TG value and is commensurate with the ability of the statin to lower LDL-C. Estrogens, which are not classed as lipid-regulating agents, may be used to lower LDL-C and increase HDL-C in some postmenopausal women (see B.3.4 and Table D.6-6). In hypertriglyceridemic women, transdermal estrogens rather than oral estrogens may be used. When opposed therapy is necessary, progesterone is preferable to medroxyprogesterone when HDL-C is low.

Table 2.9-2. Selection of Lipid-Regulating Drugs

Category	First Choices	Alternative	Combination Therapy
Hypercholesterolemia*	Statin, resin	Niacin, fibrate	Statin + resin; resin + niacin; statin + fibrate[†]
Combined hyperlipidemia	Fibrate, niacin, statin		Statin + fibrate[†]; resin + fibrate; resin + niacin; fibrate + niacin; statin + niacin[‡]
Hypertriglyceridemia	Fibrate, niacin	Statin	Fibrate + niacin

Note: For drug recommendations in adults with diabetes mellitus, see Table B.1-6.

*May also consider ERT in postmenopausal women.

†The combination of a statin and a fibrate must be used with caution because of increased risk for myopathy.

‡There is increased risk for myopathy and liver dysfunction with the combination of a statin and niacin.

Table 2.9-3. Effects of Lipid-Regulating Drug Classes on Major Plasma Lipid Values

	Statins	Resins	Niacin	Fibrates
LDL-C	↓↓↓↓	↓↓↓	↓↓	↑ or ↓↓
HDL-C	↑	0 to ↑	↑↑	↑↑
TG (VLDL)	↓ to ↓↓	0 to ↑	↓↓↓	↓↓↓

2.10 Monitor Lipid-Regulating Interventions

Lipid concentrations in patients prescribed lifestyle or pharmacologic interventions must be monitored periodically to determine the efficacy of the regimen, to serve for further counseling of the patient, and to help identify any adverse effects of therapy. There must be monitoring at all times for possible untoward drug interactions.

Table 2.10-1. Suggested Monitoring Intervals

Intervention	Short Term	Long Term
Diet	At 1 and 3 months	Quarterly, decreasing to twice a year
Drug	At 6 weeks, then at 8- to 12-week intervals through first year	At 4- to 6-month intervals

CHART 2-1. LIPID MANAGEMENT FOR PRIMARY PREVENTION OF CHD IN ADULTS—ILIB RECOMMENDATIONS

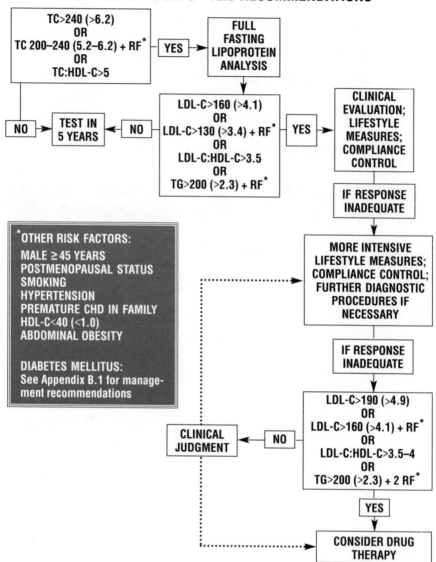

Measurement of TC alone **(minimum approach)** may be used for initial screening in patients who have no evidence of atherosclerotic disease; however, the preferred first lipid evaluation **(optimum approach)** in all patients is the full fasting lipoprotein analysis (TC, HDL-C, TG, and calculated LDL-C). CHD = coronary heart disease; HDL-C = high-density lipoprotein cholesterol; LDL-C = low-density lipoprotein cholesterol; RF = risk factor(s); TC = total cholesterol; TG = triglyceride. All lipid values are mg/dL (mmol/L). Recommended primary-prevention CHD risk calculators: **PROCAM:** www.chd-taskforce.com (interactive); **Framingham** in Wilson et al. *Circulation* 1998;97(18):1837–1847 or www.nhlbi.nih.gov/about/framingham/riskabs.htm.

CHART 2-2. LIPID MANAGEMENT FOR SECONDARY PREVENTION OF CHD IN ADULTS—ILIB RECOMMENDATIONS

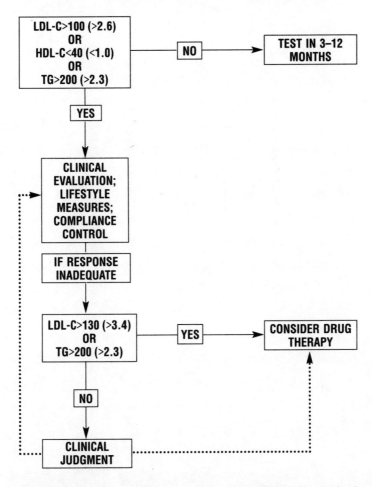

Full fasting lipoprotein analysis should always be the first lipid evaluation in patients with evidence of atherosclerotic disease. LDL-C action limits are more stringent than in primary prevention. **For management of patients with diabetes mellitus, see Appendix B.1.** HDL-C = high-density lipoprotein cholesterol; LDL-C = low-density lipoprotein cholesterol; TG = triglyceride. All lipid values are mg/dL (mmol/L).

CASE STUDIES

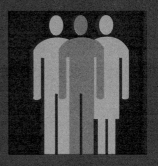

3 Case Studies

		Page
3.1. Case 1.	Elevated LDL-C in a Young Adult	75
3.2. Case 2.	Persistent Low HDL-C	77
3.3. Case 3.	Dyslipidemia and Impaired Glucose Tolerance	79
3.4. Case 4.	Dyslipidemia in Type 2 Diabetes Mellitus	81
3.5. Case 5.	Elevated LDL-C and High HDL-C	83
3.6. Case 6.	Hypercholesterolemia in a Postmenopausal Woman	85
3.7. Case 7.	Hypercholesterolemia in an Elderly Patient	87
3.8. Case 8.	Severely Elevated Plasma TG and Pancreatitis	89
3.9. Case 9.	Dyslipidemia and Established CHD	91
3.10. Case 10.	Hypercholesterolemia in Secondary Prevention	93
3.11. Case 11.	Severely Elevated LDL-C in a Young Adult	95
3.12. Case 12.	Patient with CHD, Multiple Risk Factors, and "Average" Cholesterol	97
3.13. Case 13.	Hyperlipidemia and a Family History of Premature CHD	99
3.14. Case 14.	Familial Hypercholesterolemia in a Child	101

Note: More than one answer may be correct.

Estimated 8- and 10-year absolute risks for a CHD event in the ILIB primary-prevention adult cases according to PROCAM (Münster Heart Study) and Framingham risk charts are shown in Table 3-1 on page 103. Note that the presence of a risk factor may not confer high *absolute* risk during the next 8–10 years, but will confer high risk over a lifetime of exposure. Moreover, assessments by categorical risk factors may falsely reassure individuals who are at high risk from multiple marginal abnormalities. Nevertheless, risk charts are useful in encouraging the clinician to regard overall risk. They may be used to motivate or reassure patients, and may assist in the selection of therapies. Risk charts do not replace clinical judgment and a complete clinical evaluation.

3.1 Case 1. Elevated LDL-C in a Young Adult

A 33-year-old man presented to an internist for a routine checkup. He proved to be in excellent health except for hypercholesterolemia found on fasting analysis: TC of 280 mg/dL (7.2 mmol/L), HDL-C of 60 mg/dL (1.6 mmol/L), TG of 140 mg/dL (1.6 mmol/L), and calculated LDL-C of 192 mg/dL (4.9 mmol/L). Lp[a] was 13 mg/dL. Repeat blood sampling confirmed the lipid profile. Thyroid, renal, and hepatic values were normal, and results of a glucose tolerance test were normal. Blood pressure was 110/70 mm Hg. There were no clinical manifestations of hypercholesterolemia.

Family history was negative for hypertension, diabetes mellitus, and premature CVD, and the patient described his parents and older brother as having normal lipid values. The patient had never smoked, was not overweight (173 cm and 64 kg, or 5 ft 8 in and 140 lb, BMI 21.3 kg/m²), and played vigorous singles tennis on weekends in addition to jogging 5–6 km (3–4 miles) three times a week.

The patient was advised to follow the general cholesterol-lowering diet (NCEP Step I Diet), with total fat not to exceed 30% of energy intake, saturated fat not to exceed 10% of energy intake, and no more than 300 mg/day dietary cholesterol. Lipid values were checked over a period of several months, and LDL-C stabilized at about 170 mg/dL (4.4 mmol/L). Despite referral to a dietitian, the patient was unable to comply with a more rigorous diet, which he attributed to his travel and social obligations.

What do you recommend to the patient?

A. Begin low-dose cholestyramine (8 g/day) in divided doses.

B. Begin nicotinic acid, titrated up to 1 g t.i.d.

C. Continue with the present program.

D. Begin gemfibrozil 600 mg b.i.d.

E. Begin an HMG-CoA reductase inhibitor.

Answer: C. Continue with the present program

LDL-C remained elevated (>160 mg/dL, or >4.1 mmol/L) despite exercise and maximum efforts toward dietary control. However, given the patient's relative youth, otherwise acceptable lipid profile, including high HDL-C and the absence of other risk for CHD, it would be best to defer consideration of lipid-lowering pharmacotherapy, which is usually long-term or lifelong therapy. The patient's LDL-C:HDL-C ratio (2.8) is now at a desirable level (<3) for primary prevention; still, it would be best to reduce his LDL-C to <130 mg/dL (<3.4 mmol/L). The physician should be watchful for the development of other risk factors, for example, MI in the patient's brother or calcification of the aorta, which would indicate higher risk. Lp[a] is in the desirable range (<30 mg/dL); Lp[a] concentration may provide additional risk information in some patients.

Had this same patient had another risk factor—for example, cigarette smoking, hypertension, or a family history of early CVD—lipid-lowering drug therapy as a supplement to dietary intervention would have been advisable because of the high global risk for CHD. The physician should congratulate the patient on his healthful lifestyle and encourage him to remain trim and active and not to start smoking.

If this patient has children, the physician should recommend that they undergo cholesterol screening. The NCEP Expert Panel on Blood Cholesterol Levels in Children and Adolescents recommends that choles-terol screening be performed in young people if a parent has TC ≥240 mg/dL (≥6.2 mmol/L) or if evidence of early atherosclerotic disease has been found in a parent or grandparent (see Appendix B.2 for assessment and treatment of dyslipidemia in pediatric patients). Cardiologists and other physicians who see adult patients should make a routine practice of referring the offspring of hypercholesterolemic or high-risk patients to a source of continuing health care for lipid testing and follow-up. This point should be borne in mind in following case studies as well.

3.2 Case 2. Persistent Low HDL-C

An asymptomatic 45-year-old man has sought medical advice because lipid screening at a company health fair showed his LDL-C to be moderately elevated and his HDL-C to be low. Fasting blood sampling at your office confirms dyslipidemia: TC, 195 mg/dL (5.0 mmol/L); HDL-C, 27 mg/dL (0.7 mmol/L); TG, 160 mg/dL (1.8 mmol/L); calculated LDL-C, 136 mg/dL (3.5 mmol/L). Fasting plasma glucose is 115 mg/dL (6.4 mmol/L) (impaired). The patient is 168 cm (5 ft 6 in) in height and weighs 85 kg (187 lb). His waist circumference is 96.5 cm (38 in). He is physically active but follows no special diet, and smokes about 1 pack of cigarettes per day. His blood pressure is 120/80 mm Hg. Results of physical examination and other laboratory tests are unremarkable. Family history is negative for early CVD.

Over a period of 6 months, you and your staff work with the patient to encourage him to stop smoking, lose weight, and follow an energy-restricted diet low in saturated fat, cholesterol, and sugar. The patient is able to cut his cigarette consumption by about three fourths, and he has intensified his exercise regimen. He complies strictly with the dietary guidelines except that he is unable to reduce his energy intake to achieve weight loss, reporting that his reduction in smoking precludes further restriction. Follow-up lipid assessments have shown a gradual improvement in the LDL-C and HDL-C values; the latest values are 128 mg/dL (3.3 mmol/L) and 31 mg/dL (0.8 mmol/L). The TG concentration has remained stable. Fasting glucose is now 105 mg/dL (5.8 mmol/L).

Which of the following therapeutic options is the most appropriate next step?

A. Begin a statin.

B. Begin nicotinic acid, titrated up to 1 g t.i.d.

C. Work further with the patient on lifestyle changes.

D. Advise the patient to continue with the present program and to add an alcoholic drink each day to increase his HDL-C.

Answer: C. Work further with the patient on lifestyle changes

The patient has shown excellent compliance with diet but has not been able to quit smoking or lose weight. His LDL-C value is now acceptable, probably largely because of the reduction in saturated fat, and his TG value, although slightly higher than desirable, is below the initiation concentration for intervention. He has increased his HDL-C to 31 mg/dL (0.8 mmol/L), but that is still a low value. Increasing HDL-C to 45 mg/dL (1.2 mmol/L) or higher should be a goal. Each increment of 1 mg/dL (0.03 mmol/L) in HDL-C is associated with about a 2% decrease of CHD risk in men or a 3% decrease of CHD risk in women in observational epidemiologic studies. Although the fasting glucose value is now in the normal range (see B.1.1), even a value >90 mg/dL (>5.0 mmol/L) possibly increases risk for macrovascular disease.

If not already tried, an intensive stop-smoking program should be recommended, and the use of nicotine replacement therapy should be encouraged or prescription of bupropion may be considered. Nicotine gum, nicotine spray, or bupropion may reduce in the short term the weight gain seen in about 80% of quitters. Complete abstinence from smoking may further increase HDL-C. At a BMI of 30.4 kg/m², the patient has class I obesity, which moderately increases risk for comorbidities; in addition, his risk for obesity-associated metabolic complications is increased by his abdominal obesity, roughly indicated in a (Caucasian) man by a waist circumference exceeding 94 cm (37 in).

Lipid-regulating pharmacotherapy is generally not recommended for isolated low HDL-C in primary prevention. Because LDL-C lowering, in particular with statin therapy, unequivocally yields major morbidity and mortality benefit, reduction of any LDL-C elevation is the first priority in intervening against dyslipidemia. AFCAPS/TexCAPS findings provide support for the clinical benefit of statin therapy in primary-prevention patients with only average LDL-C and reduced HDL-C concentrations. In secondary prevention, results of HIT include a 22% decrease in CHD events and an 11% decrease in all-cause mortality rate with gemfibrozil therapy in patients with HDL-C ≤40 mg/dL (≤1.0 mmol/L), LDL-C ≤140 mg/dL (≤3.6 mmol/L), and TG ≤300 mg/dL (≤3.4 mmol/L). (See Introduction for discussion of these trials.)

3.3 Case 3. Dyslipidemia and Impaired Glucose Tolerance

A 58-year-old man with impaired glucose tolerance and hypertension comes to your office with the following fasting lipid profile: TC, 250 mg/dL (6.5 mmol/L); HDL-C, 30 mg/dL (0.8 mmol/L); TG, 300 mg/dL (3.4 mmol/L); calculated LDL-C, 160 mg/dL (4.2 mmol/L). His blood pressure from measurement on three occasions averages 156/100 mm Hg; there is no evidence of target organ damage. Fasting glucose is 115 mg/dL (6.4 mmol/L); 2-hour postprandial glucose is 180 mg/dL (9.9 mmol/L). The patient, a nonsmoker and nondrinker, consumes a typical western diet and is overweight (170 cm and 86 kg, or 5 ft 7 in and 190 lb; BMI 29.8 kg/m²), with a waist:hip ratio of 1.2 and a waist circumference of 98 cm (39 in). He has a sedentary occupation and does not exercise on a regular basis.

You prescribe an ACE inhibitor and initiate dietary intervention as well as prescribe monitored, individualized increase in physical activity that takes account of the patient's low level of fitness. After 4 months of lifestyle intervention, including further restriction of saturated fat and cholesterol under a dietitian's supervision, the lipid values are very little changed: TC, 240 mg/dL (6.2 mmol/L); HDL-C, 30 mg/dL (0.8 mmol/L); TG, 283 mg/dL (3.2 mmol/L); calculated LDL-C, 153 mg/dL (4.0 mmol/L). Blood pressure has normalized (128/84 mm Hg). Fasting glucose is 111 mg/dL (6.2 mmol/L); 2-hour postprandial glucose is 130 mg/dL (7.2 mmol/L). The patient has achieved a 5.5-kg (12-lb) weight loss.

Given the patient's overall high risk for CHD, you consider it advisable to add lipid-regulating drug therapy to his regimen. Which of the following drug selections would be appropriate?

A. Nicotinic acid, titrated up to 1 g t.i.d.

B. A fibric-acid derivative

C. An HMG-CoA reductase inhibitor

D. A fibric-acid derivative plus low-dose bile-acid sequestrant

Answer: B or C. A fibric-acid derivative or an HMG-CoA reductase inhibitor

Although this patient has not yet had symptoms of atherosclerotic disease, he is at high risk from multiple risk factors for a CHD event. In terms of major risk factors, he has dyslipidemia, hypertension, and central obesity and is older than 45. Beyond the major risk factors, he is sedentary and has impaired glucose tolerance (110–125 mg/dL, or 6.1–6.9 mmol/L by ADA definitions).

In choosing to opt for lipid-regulating drug treatment at an LDL-C value of 153 mg/dL (4.0 mmol/L) and a TG value of 283 mg/dL (3.2 mmol/L), the physician is using clinical judgment about global risk. In primary prevention if other risk is present and dyslipidemia is resistant to lifestyle management, drugs are generally recommended by the ILIB at LDL-C of 160 mg/dL (4.1 mmol/L) and TG of 200 mg/dL (2.3 mmol/L).

In dyslipidemia, the patient not only has hypercholesterolemia and low HDL-C, but also is hypertriglyceridemic—a combination that has been associated in major clinical studies with very high risk. Subjects with elevated plasma TG tend to have small, dense LDL. A predominance of small, dense LDL has been associated in some prospective studies with increased risk for MI, and is more prevalent in diabetic than in nondiabetic subjects.

A fibrate would be a reasonable choice for this patient's combination of low HDL-C, moderately elevated LDL-C, and elevated TG. The minimum 15% LDL-C lowering and 30% TG lowering needed in this patient are well within the efficacy range of fibrates; in addition, fibrates typically increase HDL-C 10–30%. It is of interest that with TG lowering by a fibrate, the LDL population tends to shift from small, dense particles to large, buoyant (normal) particles. However, fibrates may have little effect on lowering elevated LDL-C when TG is elevated. An HMG-CoA reductase inhibitor could be used to lower LDL-C, and statins have beneficial effects on HDL-C and TG as well. Although nicotinic acid has favorable effects on all three major lipid fractions, it is not recommended in patients with impaired glucose tolerance because it can worsen glucose intolerance. Bile-acid resins have little effect on HDL-C concentrations and may increase TG.

3.4 Case 4. Dyslipidemia in Type 2 Diabetes Mellitus

The patient is an asymptomatic 40-year-old woman who was diagnosed with type 2 diabetes mellitus 5 years ago. She has always been mildly overweight but has remained normotensive. Physical examination shows a weight of 71 kg (156 lb) and blood pressure of 110/70 mm Hg; the patient is 165 cm (5 ft 5 in) (BMI 26.3 kg/m^2). She has never smoked. She describes her mother, who died at age 50 in an accident, as also having had "adult-onset" diabetes and as having had peripheral vascular complications. The patient's father died of an MI at age 49. She has one sibling, a half-brother who is 35 and in apparent good health, although he rarely sees a physician. She is married and has a 22-year-old daughter and an 18-year-old son, neither of whom has had any health problems; both are normoglycemic, normotensive, and normolipidemic. The patient maintains good glycemic control through scrupulous compliance with a regimen of diet, exercise, and glyburide. Her glycosylated hemoglobin is 6.5%. She does not drink and she emphasizes complex carbohydrates and fiber in her diet, but she is not a vegetarian.

The patient's lipid profile has been closely monitored for only about 1 year. Despite her good glycemic control and the inclusion of a cholesterol-lowering focus in her regimen, her fasting lipids have stabilized at average values of TC 215 (5.6), HDL-C 39 (1.0), TG 290 (3.3), and calculated LDL-C 118 (3.1), all values mg/dL (mmol/L).

Would lipid-regulating pharmacotherapy be appropriate in this patient, and, if so, which agent would be your first choice?

A. Nicotinic acid

B. An HMG-CoA reductase inhibitor

C. A fibric-acid derivative

D. A fibric-acid derivative plus low-dose bile-acid sequestrant

E. Pharmacotherapy not appropriate

Answer: B. An HMG-CoA reductase inhibitor

Although symptoms or signs of atherosclerotic disease are not present, the patient is at high lifetime risk for CHD. She has the typical dyslipidemia of type 2 diabetes, namely, elevated TG and reduced HDL-C. Type 2 diabetes increases CHD risk three to seven times in women compared with two to three times in men. It nearly eliminates any female pre-menopausal cardioprotection, and there is evidence that plasma TG and HDL-C are stronger risk predictors in women than men.

The slight elevation in the patient's TC would largely represent the cholesterol carried in VLDL particles. Nevertheless, the LDL-C value is above the goal of 100 mg/dL (2.6 mmol/L) or less in diabetic subjects. Lipid-regulating drug intervention is recommended by the ADA and the ILIB at 130 mg/dL (3.4 mmol/L), but may be appropriate in cases of high risk when values fall between 100 mg/dL and 130 mg/dL. The ILIB recommends consideration of drug therapy when TG remains >400 mg/dL (>4.6 mmol/L) in the absence of other risk, or >200 mg/dL (>2.3 mmol/L) with one or more other major risk factors present in primary-prevention diabetic patients. If macrovascular disease is present, drugs should be considered if there is persistent LDL-C >100 mg/dL (>2.6 mmol/L) or persistent TG >150 mg/dL (>1.7 mmol/L).

The ADA recommends statins as first-choice lipid-regulating pharmacotherapy (after improved glycemic control) in diabetic patients with combined hyperlipidemia. Statin therapy typically reduces LDL-C by 15–60% and increases HDL-C by 5–10%, although individual response can be variable. Typical reductions in plasma TG range from 10% to 20%, although in HTG atorvastatin has reduced TG 26–46%. Good evidence to support significant reductions in CVD clinical event rates (including both coronary and cerebrovascular events) in diabetic patients is available from subset analyses of large, long-term statin trials (see B.1.3.1).

The ADA's second choice in combined hyperlipidemia is improved glycemic control plus a statin plus a fibrate. Fibrates are excellent drugs for lowering TG and raising HDL-C.

Third-choice lipid-regulating pharmacotherapy in the ADA guidelines is improved glycemic control plus a resin plus a fibrate, or improved glycemic control plus a statin plus nicotinic acid.

3.5 Case 5. Elevated LDL-C and High HDL-C

An asymptomatic 45-year-old woman wants your advice about her cholesterol concentration, which was originally found to be severely elevated (320 mg/dL, or 8.3 mmol/L) by desktop analysis at a health fair 3 months ago. On the basis of literature from the fair, the patient began the intensified cholesterol-lowering diet (25–27% of energy as fat, 6–8% of energy as saturated fat, cholesterol <200–250 mg/day). She had already been following a decreased-fat, low-sodium diet, in part because of a history of hypertension. A week ago, the patient was disappointed to learn from a fingerstick cholesterol test at the pharmacy that her TC, although reduced somewhat, had not normalized.

Your fasting lipoprotein analysis shows TC 293, HDL-C 85, TG 142, and calculated LDL-C 180 in mg/dL, or TC 7.6, HDL-C 2.2, TG 1.6, and LDL-C 4.7 in mmol/L. The patient is taking an ACE inhibitor and blood pressure has been normalized (105/70 mm Hg). She has no history of diabetes mellitus and is premenopausal. She does not smoke, and drinks an occasional cocktail. She is 160 cm (5 ft 3 in) in height and weighs 56 kg (123 lb) (BMI 21.9 kg/m^2); she appears quite fit. She has always been physically active; currently, she attends a weekly aerobic exercise class, plays tennis once a week, and walks briskly for about 45 minutes on Saturday and on Sunday. In regard to her low-fat diet, she characterizes herself as "more than a bean counter—a milligram counter." Physical examination is unremarkable, and thyroid-stimulating hormone and other laboratory values are normal. Family history is not significant except for hypertension in her mother.

What do you recommend to the patient?

A. Continue the healthful lifestyle.

B. Begin a bile-acid sequestrant.

C. Begin an HMG-CoA reductase inhibitor.

D. Begin nicotinic acid.

Answer: A. Continue the healthful lifestyle

Lipid-regulating pharmacotherapy should be considered in primary prevention if after dietary intervention LDL-C remains >160 mg/dL (>4.1 mmol/L) and there is other major risk for CHD. This patient has LDL-C of 180 mg/dL (4.7 mmol/L) despite a long-standing healthful lifestyle, and she is taking antihypertensive medication (an ACE inhibitor, which would have little if any effect on lipid concentrations—see Table D.6-8). She has an HDL-C value of 85 mg/dL (2.2 mmol/L), and high HDL-C affords a degree of cardioprotection. Concern is also lessened because the patient's TC:HDL-C ratio (3.4) is well below 4.5 and her LDL-C:HDL-C ratio (2.1) is well below 3; TC:HDL-C <4.5 and LDL-C:HDL-C <3 are useful goals in primary prevention.

Further, the patient has the relative protection against CHD conferred by premenopausal status. That the patient is fit and has an acceptable BMI also improves the global risk profile. Continuation of a healthful lifestyle and reevaluation, including a lipoprotein profile, at least within 1 year would be the best option. It would be advisable for the patient to consult a dietitian to confirm that her dietary intake conforms with the intensified cholesterol-lowering diet. The physician needs to reassure the patient—to help her understand how her lipid profile fits into her global CHD risk profile, and to support her excellent health habits.

3.6 Case 6. Hypercholesterolemia in a Postmenopausal Woman

An asymptomatic attorney consults you near the time of her 55th birthday for assessment of her CVD risk status. She is concerned because her mother died of an MI at age 55. She is taking no medications, does not smoke, and is not overweight (165 cm and 64 kg, or 5 ft 5 in and 140 lb; BMI 23.5 kg/m²) although she is sedentary. She follows no special diet and reports she takes an occasional mixed drink at parties or wine with dinner. Blood pressure is 120/80 mm Hg. Her fasting lipoprotein profile is TC 240 mg/dL (6.2 mmol/L), HDL-C 40 mg/dL (1.0 mmol/L), TG 100 mg/dL (1.1 mmol/L), and calculated LDL-C 180 mg/dL (4.7 mmol/L). Other physical examination and routine laboratory findings are normal. Bone density measured in the lumbar spine is normal (1.20 g/cm²).

You instruct the patient in the cholesterol-lowering diet and outline an exercise regimen. At 3 months, there is essentially no change in the lipid profile, and the patient reports that she has not increased her physical activity or heeded the diet. Upon referral to a dietitian, the patient makes some commitment to the cholesterol-lowering regimen; at 8 months after presentation the profile is TC 219, HDL-C 41, TG 110, and calculated LDL-C 156 in mg/dL, or TC 5.7, HDL-C 1.1, TG 1.2, and LDL-C 4.1 in mmol/L, very similar to recent interim values.

The dietitian has advised you that although she will keep encouraging the patient, she believes maximum compliance may have been achieved.

You decide to initiate treatment in addition to lifestyle intervention. Which of the following would be the best choice for this patient?

A. Conjugated estrogen, 0.625 mg/day

B. Nicotinic acid, titrated up to 1 g t.i.d., with meals

C. A fibric-acid derivative

D. An HMG-CoA reductase inhibitor

E. Bile-acid sequestrant in divided doses

Answer: D. An HMG-CoA reductase inhibitor

The patient is at high lifetime risk for CHD because of multiple major risk factors. With what is probably maximum dietary compliance in this case, the elevated LDL-C has decreased by 13% and HDL-C has changed very little. LDL-C no higher than 130 mg/dL (3.4 mmol/L)—and preferably a lower LDL-C value—should be achieved, and a higher HDL-C concentration would be advisable. A statin at a low dosage would be a good choice to lower the LDL-C effectively, and this class of agents has excellent tolerability and safety. A moderate increase in HDL-C and a moderate decrease in plasma TG would also be expected. Subset analyses now available from large, randomized trials of statins show the clinical benefit of aggressive cholesterol-lowering therapy in women to equal or even exceed that in men. Risk for a first major coronary event was reduced 46% in the postmenopausal, generally healthy women of AFCAPS/TexCAPS, compared with 37% in the men in that primary-prevention trial of lovastatin (Downs et al. JAMA 1998;279:1615–1622). Like this patient, AFCAPS/TexCAPS patients had only average cholesterol concentrations and below-average HDL-C. Statin therapy in women who already have established CHD has achieved reductions in a variety of CVD events, including fatal and nonfatal MI, coronary revascularization procedures, and stroke.

Another possible, although controversial, option for the management of dyslipidemia in the patient would be ERT. In postmenopausal women, orally administered estrogen decreases LDL-C by about 15% and increases HDL-C by about the same amount. Thus, estrogen replacement might be able to achieve the minimum lipid goals in this case. Estrogen replacement would not need to be supplemented with a progestin because of the hysterectomy.

It should be noted that estrogen does not have a U.S. Food and Drug Administration indication for either lipid regulation or reduction of CHD risk. Observational epidemiologic data support the concept, but data from large, randomized prospective trials are lacking except for those from HERS. In HERS, a trial in women with established CHD, risk for nonfatal MI or CHD death increased during the first year of estrogen–progestin therapy. Therefore, it does not appear advisable to start combination hormone-replacement therapy de novo in women with CHD.

3.7 Case 7. Hypercholesterolemia in an Elderly Patient

A 74-year-old man has been referred to your office for further evaluation of hyperlipidemia. He has a history of hypertension treated with an ACE inhibitor (current blood pressure 130/80 mm Hg) but is otherwise without complaint; other laboratory tests, including thyroid-stimulating hormone measurement, are normal. He is 170 cm (5 ft 7 in) in height and weighs 68 kg (150 lb) (BMI 23.5 kg/m^2), does not smoke, and walks approximately 3 km (2 miles) four times a week. His father died of a stroke at age 52, and a sister had coronary artery bypass surgery at age 60. Six months ago, the patient had a fasting lipoprotein analysis, which yielded the following results: TC 278, HDL-C 38, TG 133, and calculated LDL-C 213 in mg/dL, or TC 7.2, HDL-C 1.0, TG 1.5, and LDL-C 5.5 in mmol/L. He was referred to a dietitian, who placed him on the cholesterol-lowering diet. The diet was intensified after 2 months because of inadequate LDL-C response. Repeat lipoprotein profile 1 week ago yielded values of TC 250, HDL-C 40, TG 90, and calculated LDL-C 192 in mg/dL, or TC 6.5, HDL-C 1.0, TG 1.0, and LDL-C 5.0 in mmol/L, consonant with recent interim values.

The most appropriate lipid-regulating pharmacologic therapy would be:

A.   A bile-acid sequestrant at a low dose

B.   A fibric-acid derivative

C.   Nicotinic acid, titrated up to 1 g t.i.d., with meals

D.   An HMG-CoA reductase inhibitor

Answer: D. An HMG-CoA reductase inhibitor

The patient is at high risk for CHD because of the presence of multiple risk factors: his age, hypercholesterolemia, hypertension, and family history of early CVD. Absolute risk for CVD morbidity and mortality rises steeply with age, and major risk factors continue to operate beyond age 60 and even beyond age 70. High-risk but otherwise healthy elderly patients are candidates for lipid-lowering therapy, including drug therapy.

Potential side effects must be considered with particular care in the elderly. Both statins and fibrates are well tolerated in older patients. In this case, LDL-C lowering is needed, so a statin would be appropriate, begun at a low dosage. The LDL-C goal in primary prevention is <130 mg/dL (<3.4 mmol/L); thus, LDL-C needs to be lowered at least 30%. Although additional clinical trial data in the elderly are needed for full support of drug treatment, subgroup analyses of the recent statin clinical endpoint trials support lipid lowering in both primary prevention (WOSCOPS, AFCAPS/TexCAPS) and secondary prevention (4S, CARE, LIPID) in older and elderly patients (see Appendix B.4). Statin therapy was well tolerated by elderly patients in the trials, with remarkably low rates of adverse effects. In 4S and CARE, absolute risk reduction with statin therapy was approximately doubled in older patients compared with younger patients. Some data support enhanced response to statin therapy with increasing age. Trials designed to assess clinical outcomes of lipid-regulating therapy in the elderly are ongoing, for example, the Prospective Study of Pravastatin in the Elderly at Risk (PROSPER), the Fluvastatin Assessment of Morbidity/Mortality in the Elderly (FAME) study, and, including large numbers of elderly patients, the Medical Research Council/British Heart Foundation Heart Protection Study.

In the elderly, hypothyroidism is a common underlying cause of dyslipidemia and often entails few symptoms. Hypothyroidism chiefly causes LDL-C elevation; any patient with LDL-C >190 mg/dL (>4.9 mmol/L) should be tested for reduced thyroid function.

3.8 Case 8. Severely Elevated Plasma TG and Pancreatitis

An obese 40-year-old woman is referred to you after an episode of pancreatitis. She is sedentary and denies use of alcohol or tobacco. Five years ago, she was found to have impaired glucose tolerance and was advised to lose weight. She did not lose weight, and she remained in her usual state of health until 2 months ago, when she experienced midabdominal pain after a fatty meal. Evaluation at the hospital revealed elevated amylase and lipase values. Serum carbohydrate-deficient transferrin, gamma-glutamyltransferase, and uric acid values were normal. Abdominal ultrasound showed no gallstones. She gradually recovered from the pancreatitis.

Her fasting lipid profile at presentation is TG 2,500 mg/dL (28.2 mmol/L) and TC 500 mg/dL (12.9 mmol/L). A plasma sample refrigerated overnight shows a creamy supernatant and turbid infranatant. The patient's physical examination findings are unchanged except that her abdomen is now nontender and a vascular spider (spider angioma) is detected. Blood pressure is 100/70 mm Hg, and the patient is taking no drugs except ibuprofen. Fasting blood glucose is 125 mg/dL (6.9 mmol/L). The patient, with a BMI of 41.0 kg/m^2, is extremely obese (obesity class III); she is 163 cm (5 ft 4 in) in height and weighs 109 kg (240 lb), and her waist circumference is 112 cm (44 in). Her family history is negative for obesity, hypertension, diabetes mellitus, and early CVD. After intensive dietary intervention (a liquid diet), TG stabilizes at between 1,000 and 1,200 mg/dL (11.3–13.5 mmol/L).

Which lipid-regulating drug(s) would be appropriate in this patient?

A. Low-dose cholestyramine (8 g/day) in divided doses

B. Nicotinic acid t.i.d., titrated up to 1 g/day

C. A fibric-acid derivative

D. An HMG-CoA reductase inhibitor

Answer: C. A fibric-acid derivative

Therapy should be targeted toward the severe HTG. Pancreatitis is a life-threatening condition and aggressive intervention is required. Nicotinic acid lowers TG 20–50% but tends to worsen glycemic control and can lead to overt diabetes in a patient with glucose intolerance. Fibric-acid derivatives decrease TG 20–60%. If TG <500 mg/dL (<5.6 mmol/L) is achieved, therapy should be considered successful, because TG concentrations are infrequently normalized in patients with severely elevated TG.

It is imperative that this patient lose weight, and the fasting glucose value should rapidly improve with weight loss. She needs to follow an energy-restricted, low-fat diet (<20% of energy intake as total fat), and she should be placed on such a diet under the supervision of a dietitian, with close medical and dietary monitoring. In addition, the patient needs gradually to begin an exercise program under medical supervision; the exercise needs to be individualized to her low level of fitness.

If adequate TG reduction is not achieved, capsules of fish oil derived from muscle (not liver) may be added. A suitable initial dosage provides 1.5 g eicosapentaenoic acid plus docosahexaenoic acid (omega-3 fatty acids) twice daily. The TG-lowering effects of fish oils (typically, decreases of 25–30%) appear to be sustainable as long as therapeutic dosages are given.

Potential side effects of fish oil supplementation include nosebleeds, easy bruising, and GI upsets. Products that are not well refined may contain pesticides and heavy metals. With some preparations there is vitamin A and vitamin D toxicity. Fish oils may be difficult to take because of a fishy odor, although highly purified forms offer benefit in this regard.

CHD risk:benefit of fish oil supplementation is not established, although many beneficial nonlipid effects have been posited, for example, anti-inflammatory effects, an improved coagulation profile, and, in hypertensive individuals, small decreases in blood pressure. There is increasing evidence that omega-3 fatty acids have a strong antiarrhythmic effect.

3.9 Case 9. Dyslipidemia and Established CHD

A 62-year-old man underwent two-vessel CABG 3 months ago subsequent to angina and demonstration of severe stenosis. He has made an excellent recovery from the surgery. He is mildly overweight (175 cm and 83 kg, or 5 ft 9 in and 184 lb; BMI 26.8 kg/m², waist circumference 90 cm, or 35 in) and has a history of hypertension controlled by an ACE inhibitor (current blood pressure 130/80 mm Hg). He has never smoked and occasionally drinks a beer or two. He eats at restaurants almost daily and does not take any regular exercise. His family history is negative for hypertension, diabetes mellitus, and premature CVD. The fasting lipid profile is TC 206, HDL-C 23, TG 292, and calculated LDL-C 125 in mg/dL, or TC 5.3, HDL-C 0.6, TG 3.3, and LDL-C 3.2 in mmol/L. A repeat lipoprotein profile 10 days later yields similar results.

Under the supervision of a dietitian, the patient begins the intensified cholesterol-lowering diet. The dietitian includes emphasis on complex carbohydrates and raising the ratio of monounsaturated to saturated fatty acids because of the HTG. She guides the patient in the selection of restaurant foods and encourages home preparation of meals. The patient also begins a medically supervised program of daily walking.

After 6 weeks of lifestyle intervention, the confirmed fasting lipid profile is TC 207, HDL-C 29, TG 290, and calculated LDL-C 120 in mg/dL, or TC 5.3, HDL-C 0.7, TG 3.3, and LDL-C 3.1 in mmol/L.

Lipid-regulating pharmacologic management added to the supervised lifestyle interventions would preferably be in the form of:

A.   Low-dose cholestyramine (8 g/day) in divided doses

B.   Nicotinic acid, titrated up to 1 g t.i.d.

C.   A fibric-acid derivative

D.   An HMG-CoA reductase inhibitor

Answer: D. An HMG-CoA reductase inhibitor

All patients with established CHD are at very high risk for a coronary event. Aggressive LDL-C reduction is now considered mandatory in secondary-prevention patients in whom LDL-C exceeds 100 mg/dL (2.6 mmol/L). Had the initial LDL-C value been 130 mg/dL (3.4 mmol/L) or higher, the physician may have chosen to begin lipid-regulating pharmacotherapy and lifestyle changes simultaneously, as recommended by a task force of the American Heart Association (Grundy et al. Circulation 1997;95:1683–1685). That option may also be chosen according to clinical judgment when LDL-C falls between 100 and 130 mg/dL (2.6–3.4 mmol/L).

Although the patient has low HDL-C and elevated TG, the priority for lipid management is his still-elevated LDL-C, which should be reduced to below 100 mg/dL (2.6 mmol/L). Results of the 4S, CARE, LIPID, and AVERT statin trials (see 1.5.2) have erased any doubts about the value of aggressive cholesterol-lowering therapy as secondary prevention. The trial results demonstrated not only reduction of CHD events, including MI, CHD death, and revascularization procedures, but also reduction of all-cause mortality rate and stroke.

In addition, statin therapy has been shown in a number of angiographically monitored trials to reduce the progression of coronary atherosclerosis, including in patients without high LDL-C (e.g., LCAS). The Post-CABG trial assessed the effects of lipid lowering with lovastatin on saphenous vein grafts. The patients in whom LDL-C was lowered to a range of 93 to 97 mg/dL (2.4–2.5 mmol/L) by aggressive treatment did significantly better than those who achieved LDL-C in the range of 132 to 136 mg/dL (3.4–3.5 mmol/L) with moderate treatment. At the study's end, 27% of patients in the aggressive treatment group has lesion progression in grafts, compared with 39% of patients receiving moderate treatment.

Evidence to support clinical benefit of fibrate use must be considered slight at this time compared with the strong proof of morbidity and mortality reductions with statins. A fibrate might also be combined with a statin were HDL-C and TG effects of the statin inadequate. The patient should be warned about and carefully monitored for myopathic complications with this combination. The exact mechanism for the fibrate–statin interaction, which appears to be uncommon (1% of patients in a review of clinical trials), is unknown.

3.10 Case 10. Hypercholesterolemia in Secondary Prevention

A 62-year-old man presents for lipid reassessment 3 months after an inferior wall MI. During hospitalization for the MI, he had been started on an HMG-CoA reductase inhibitor at a low dosage as well as once-daily aspirin. He was also prescribed the intensified cholesterol-lowering diet (Step II Diet), implemented under the supervision of a dietitian, and moderate exercise, undertaken as part of a medically supervised cardiac rehabilitation program. His lipid values, determined from a blood sample taken within a few hours of his hospital admission for the MI, were TC 251 mg/dL (6.5 mmol/L), HDL-C 40 mg/dL (1.0 mmol/L), TG 168 mg/dL (1.9 mmol/L), and calculated LDL-C 177 mg/dL (4.6 mmol/L).

The patient had been a cigarette smoker for 30 years, but quit smoking after his hospitalization. He has no history of hypertension or diabetes mellitus. He is 173 cm (5 ft 8 in) in height and weighs 73 kg (160 lb), values yielding a BMI of 24.4 kg/m². His waist circumference is 88 cm (35 in). Blood pressure is 130/80 mm Hg. His family history includes a nonfatal heart attack in his mother when she was about age 60. He reports that he has been taking his medications regularly and that he feels he has good compliance with the lifestyle changes. The mainstay of his exercise regimen is daily walking. The current lipid profile is TC 203, HDL-C 45, TG 140, and calculated LDL-C 130 in mg/dL, or TC 5.3, HDL-C 1.2, TG 1.6, and LDL-C 3.4 in mmol/L.

What is the next therapeutic step for lipid management?

A. Increase the dosage of the statin.

B. Add a fibric-acid derivative.

C. Add nicotinic acid.

D. Add a bile-acid sequestrant.

E. Intensify dietary intervention.

Answer: A or D. Increase the dosage of the statin or add a bile-acid sequestrant

The highest risk for an atherosclerotic event is in patients who have already had an event, and the most aggressive cholesterol-lowering therapy is recommended for these patients. LDL-C in this MI survivor remains elevated at 130 mg/dL (3.4 mmol/L) and should be reduced to below 100 mg/dL (2.6 mmol/L).

An increased dosage of the statin could be tried. Atorvastatin has been reported to have greater efficacy in LDL-C reduction than milligram-equivalent doses of (in descending order) simvastatin, pravastatin, lovastatin, or fluvastatin (Jones et al. for the CURVES Investigators Am J Cardiol 1998;81:582–587). As monotherapy, it reduces LDL-C up to 60%. The 40–50% reduction needed from the initial value should be easily obtained by 40 mg/day atorvastatin.

Although meta-analyses have indicated that the CHD and total mortality risk reductions with statins can be attributed to their cholesterol-lowering effect and appear to be largely related to the degree to which they lower cholesterol (Bucher et al. Arterioscler Thromb Vasc Biol 1999;19:187–195; Gould et al. Circulation 1998;97:946–952), data are needed from randomized clinical trials designed to address formally whether "lower is better." The question is being addressed in secondary prevention by the 5-year Treating to New Targets (TNT) trial, using two dosages of atorvastatin (10 and 80 mg/day), and by the 5.5-year Incremental Decrease in Endpoints through Aggressive Lipid Lowering (IDEAL) trial, using atorvastatin (80 mg/day) and simvastatin (20–40 mg/day). Until results are available, guidelines should be followed that aim for LDL-C below 100 mg/dL (2.6 mmol/L). Another option would be to combine the statin with a resin. The patient has an acceptable TG concentration, so a resin is appropriate, and the statins and the resins combine well.

Note that LDL-C concentrations decrease after an MI for up to 12 weeks. Lipid concentrations should be determined within 24 (preferably 12) hours of the onset of chest pain; thereafter, definitive lipid determination should be deferred for 4–6 weeks.

3.11 Case 11. Severely Elevated LDL-C in a Young Adult

An asymptomatic 22-year-old man presents because of a strong family history of premature CHD and hypercholesterolemia. His father had triple CABG at age 46 and has TC of 400 mg/dL (10.3 mmol/L). His brother is normolipidemic, but his sister has had TC as high as 500 mg/dL (12.9 mmol/L). The patient, who is athletic, has a BMI of 23.2 kg/m^2; he is 185 cm (6 ft 1 in) in height and weighs 79 kg (174 lb). His blood pressure is 110/80 mm Hg. He does not smoke. Fasting blood sampling shows TC of 385 mg/dL (10.0 mmol/L), HDL-C of 48 mg/dL (1.2 mmol/L), TG of 85 mg/dL (1.0 mmol/L), and calculated LDL-C of 320 mg/dL (8.3 mmol/L), values confirmed by repeat testing. Tendon xanthomas are absent.

You institute a cholesterol-lowering diet, but after 12 weeks of carefully monitored therapy the LDL-C value has been reduced by only 5%. Current fasting lipid values are TC 370, HDL-C 49, TG 87, and calculated LDL-C 304 in mg/dL, or TC 9.6, HDL-C 1.3, TG 1.0, and LDL-C 7.8 in mmol/L.

Is consideration of drug therapy appropriate in this patient at this juncture?

A. No, because the patient's youth confers cardioprotection

B. No, because the only risk factor present other than hyper-cholesterolemia is a positive family history

C. No, because the dietary trial should last at least 6 months

D. Yes, because LDL-C remains very high despite dietary intervention

Answer: D. Yes, because LDL-C remains very high despite dietary intervention

The patient has high global lifetime risk for CHD because of the presence of one risk factor of severe degree. The severely elevated LDL-C and family history suggest heterozygous familial hypercholesterolemia (FH), which confers high risk for premature CHD. Drug therapy is generally required in addition to dietary intervention to lower LDL-C concentrations adequately in heterozygous FH. Patients may respond to single-agent drug therapy consisting of a statin, bile-acid resin, or nicotinic acid, or binary or even ternary drug therapy may be needed.

The physician may wish to assess carotid and femoral intima–media thickness by B-mode ultrasound to estimate "atherosclerotic burden." Because the frequency of sudden death is high in individuals with FH, some centers advocate assessment for myocardial perfusion defects through exercise thallium-201 imaging and exercise technetium-99m sestamibi (MIBI) single-photon emission computed tomography even when patients are asymptomatic.

In this patient, LDL-C needs to be reduced at least 50%. The HMG-CoA reductase inhibitors have the greatest LDL-lowering capability, and an agent in this class may be tried first, in particular because of the excellent tolerability. Atorvastatin as monotherapy may reduce LDL-C up to 60%; a 54% decrease on average in a series of patients with FH has been reported (Naoumova et al. Atherosclerosis 1996;119:203–213). When addition of an agent to a statin is needed for greater LDL-C reduction, a bile-acid resin is a good choice, and LDL-lowering success with the statin may encourage the patient to accept the side effects of the resin. Therapy should be maximal, but compatible with daily life. Atorvastatin 80 mg at bedtime plus 2 packets or scoopfuls (8 g) of cholestyramine in orange juice at lunchtime yields a >60% reduction in LDL-C and is often very well tolerated.

In the angiographically monitored University of California, San Francisco, Arteriosclerosis Specialized Center of Research (UCSF-SCOR) Intervention Trial (Kane et al. JAMA 1990;264:3007–3012), the per-patient change in percent stenosis of coronary lesions indicated regression in the group of patients with heterozygous FH treated aggressively with drugs.

3.12 Case 12. Patient with CHD, Multiple Risk Factors, and "Average" Cholesterol

A 57-year-old, postmenopausal woman was diagnosed with CHD 2 years ago, at which time she underwent angioplasty of a right coronary artery lesion. The patient's blood pressure is 138/86 mm Hg and she is over-weight at a BMI of 27.5 kg/m^2 (height 168 cm, or 5 ft 6 in; weight 77 kg, or 170 lb). Her waist circumference is 91 cm (36 in). The fasting plasma glucose value is 93 mg/dL (5.2 mmol/L). The patient reports that she does not smoke and drinks a couple of glasses of wine several evenings a week. She believes that she watches her diet fairly well, and she occasionally goes for a walk. Her mean fasting TC and calculated LDL-C concentrations are 216 and 142 mg/dL (5.6 and 3.7 mmol/L). HDL-C is 47 mg/dL (1.2 mmol/L) and TG is 135 mg/dL (1.5 mmol/L).

Because of the patient's high risk for another CHD event, you prescribe lipid-regulating drug therapy in addition to nonpharmacologic interven-tions targeting the increased blood pressure, dyslipidemia, overweight, and sedentary lifestyle. Which drug class or classes would be optimal to begin lipid-regulating therapy?

A.   HMG-CoA reductase inhibitor

B.   Nicotinic acid

C.   Bile-acid sequestrant

D.   Fibric-acid derivative

E.   HMG-CoA reductase inhibitor plus fibric-acid derivative

F.   Bile-acid sequestrant plus fibric-acid derivative

Answer: A. HMG-CoA reductase inhibitor

Given her multiple risk factors, the patient is at high lifetime risk for an MI or other CHD event. Risk reduction should be aggressive. Dietary intervention, preferably under the guidance of a dietitian, should be intensified. A regular exercise program should be substituted for the patient's desultory efforts.

Patients with established CHD or other atherosclerotic disease are candidates for lipid-lowering drug therapy when LDL-C remains 130 mg/dL (3.4 mmol/L) or higher, or above 100 mg/dL (2.6 mmol/L) if, in the physician's judgment, the patient's risk profile is sufficiently high. The trial of lifestyle changes alone may be short in patients at such high risk, or the physician may choose to begin lifestyle changes and lipid-lowering drug therapy simultaneously, including beginning lipid-lowering drug therapy before discharge in hospitalized patients.

Optimal choice for drug therapy in this patient would be a statin, which would effectively reduce her elevated LDL-C and moderately increase her fairly low HDL-C. To reach the goal of 100 mg/dL (2.6 mmol/L) or lower, the patient's LDL-C needs to be reduced 30%, which is easily within the range of statin effectiveness.

Use of a statin in MI survivors who had TC below 240 mg/dL (6.2 mmol/L) yielded significant reductions in risk for CHD and stroke in the CARE trial. The mean TC concentration among the men and women in CARE was only 209 mg/dL (5.4 mmol/L), which is nearly the same as the mean cholesterol of 206 mg/dL (5.3 mmol/L) in the U.S. adult population according to 1988–1991 findings from the National Health and Nutrition Examination Surveys (Johnson et al. JAMA 1993;269:3002–3008). In the CARE drug group, LDL-C was reduced from a mean of 139 mg/dL (3.6 mmol/L) to a mean of 97 mg/dL (2.5 mmol/L). CHD risk reduction was 46% in the women in CARE, compared with 20% in the trial's men. In the LIPID trial in men and women with CHD and a wide range of cholesterol values at baseline, statin therapy significantly reduced risk for CHD, stroke, and all-cause death, including a significant reduction of CHD risk in patients whose TC was initially <213 mg/dL (<5.5 mmol/L).

3.13 Case 13. Hyperlipidemia and a Family History of Premature CHD

A 45-year-old, premenopausal woman consults a physician after her 49-year-old brother died unexpectedly of an MI. The patient understood that her brother had high blood cholesterol, and she believes that her remaining sibling, a 42-year-old brother, has high TG but normal cholesterol. The patient's blood pressure (110/70 mm Hg) and weight (BMI 22 kg/m^2) are normal, and she has neither diabetes nor impaired glucose tolerance. She reports that she takes regular exercise, smokes several cigarettes each day, and drinks on the rare occasion and only moderately. Her father, a non-smoker, had a fatal heart attack at age 53. The patient's mean TC and calculated LDL-C are 336 mg/dL (8.7 mmol/L) and 210 mg/dL (5.4 mmol/L). Her HDL-C is 48 mg/dL (1.2 mmol/L) and her fasting TG value is 390 mg/dL (4.4 mmol/L). There are no xanthomas or corneal arcus.

Which familial lipid disorder seems most likely given the information available about the patient's lipid values and family history?

A. Heterozygous familial hypercholesterolemia

B. Familial combined hyperlipidemia

C. Dysbetalipoproteinemia

D. Familial endogenous hypertriglyceridemia

Answer: B. Familial combined hyperlipidemia

A genetic lipid disorder seems likely because both the patient's father and brother suffered early deaths from CHD and because of the family history of hyperlipidemia. A family history of premature CHD, defined by the NCEP as MI or sudden death before age 55 years in a first-degree male relative or before age 65 years in a first-degree female relative, is a major coronary risk factor.

The full clinical evaluation should include efforts to determine whether the combined hyperlipidemia is secondary or primary and should include a complete evaluation of risk factor and cardiovascular status. Family testing is essential to the diagnosis of familial disorders, and family history should include history not only of cardiovascular disease but also of dyslipidemia, hypertension, diabetes, and obesity. An important aspect of the physical examination is searching for manifestations of atherosclerosis (e.g., vascular bruits, reduced peripheral pulses), manifestations of dyslipidemia (e.g., corneal arcus, xanthomas, hepatosplenomegaly), and evidence of thyroid abnormalities.

On the basis of the lipid profile and available family history, it appears that the patient most likely has FCH, which has a prevalence of about 1% in the general population. Specific diagnostic criteria for FCH are not firmly established. Generally, a diagnosis is accepted if there is a strong family history of hyperlipidemia and early coronary disease, and the index patient and a first-degree relative have hyperlipidemia of Fredrickson phenotype IIa, IIb, or IV. All three phenotypes may be seen within a family, and the pattern may change within an individual. The absence of affected children and the absence of xanthomas are useful clinical findings; the diagnosis of FCH is typically one of adulthood. Although not the case in this patient, patients with FCH are often overweight and hypertensive, and may be diabetic and have gout. When hypercholesterolemia is present, TC is usually between 250 and 350 mg/dL (6.5–9.0 mmol/L). When HTG is present, it is usually mild to moderate, although TG elevation may be severe.

The fundamental basis of FCH, which was first described in families of survivors of premature MI, is unknown.

3.14 Case 14. Familial Hypercholesterolemia in a Child

A 9-1/2-year-old boy referred for lipid testing because of a strong family history of hypercholesterolemia and premature CHD was found to have fasting lipid values of TC 352, HDL-C 53, TG 146, and LDL-C 270 in mg/dL, or TC 9.1, HDL-C 1.4, TG 1.6, and LDL-C 7.0 in mmol/L. His maternal aunt was known to have heterozygous FH and underwent CABG at age 37. His mother, aged 44, had TC values of about 400 mg/dL (10.3 mmol/L), brought down to the low 200s (5.7–5.9 mmol/L) by lifestyle and statin therapy. His maternal grandfather, known to have tendinous xanthomas and severe hypercholesterolemia, had an MI at age 40. The patient's 14-year-old brother and 48-year-old father had normal lipid values. The patient had no significant medical history and because of his mother's hypercholesterolemia ate a fairly low fat diet, including little intake of high-fat snack foods or fast foods. His weight and blood pressure were normal, and he was physically active both at home and at school. Physical examination was negative for corneal arcus, xanthelasma, tendinous or tuberous xanthomas, and thyromegaly. Cardiac examination was normal.

The patient was a heterozygote for FH. After a 6-month trial of a carefully formulated and monitored diet with further fat restriction, the patient's lipid values were little changed; the average LDL-C was reduced by about 5%. The parents, after detailed discussion, understood that the child would need long-term therapy. They opted to add drug therapy now, rather than wait until after puberty. Which drug therapy would be advisable, and supported by NCEP guidelines?

A. Crystalline nicotinic acid, beginning at 100 mg t.i.d.
B. Extended-release nicotinic acid, beginning at 375 mg once daily
C. A bile-acid sequestrant, beginning at 2 g/day
D. A statin, beginning at a low dosage
E. None of the above: current guidelines do not support use of lipid-lowering drug therapy in children

Answer: C. A bile-acid sequestrant, beginning at 2 g/day

The NCEP pediatric guidelines recommend consideration of lipid-lowering pharmacotherapy in children ≥10 years of age when despite maximal lifestyle therapy LDL-C remains >190 mg/dL (>4.9 mmol/L) or, in the presence of multiple risk factors or a family history of premature CVD, >160 mg/dL (>4.1 mmol/L). The NCEP notes that drug therapy may be warranted in younger patients when hyperlipidemia is severe. Whether the development of atherosclerosis will be averted if aggressive therapy is withheld until age 10 or 20 years is unknown, but beginning therapy early may help prevent disease. While the LDL-C goal in the NCEP pediatric guidelines is a value <130 mg/dL (<3.4 mmol/L), the physician may wish to strive for a reasonable percentage reduction rather than for normalization in children and adolescents, deferring the most aggressive therapy until adulthood.

Because bile-acid resins have little or no systemic toxicity, they are the only lipid-lowering drugs generally recommended for use in children. They are effective and appear to be well tolerated and safe in children, although compliance may be low because of unpalatability. Low dosages are preferred and vitamin supplementation is prudent. There is diminishing cholesterol reduction with dosages beyond 8 g/day. In a 1-year, placebo-controlled, randomized trial in 96 boys and girls aged 6–11 years with FH, Tonstad et al. (J Pediatr 1996;129:42–49) found cholestyramine 8 g/day to achieve LDL-C reductions of 17–19%. Growth was not adversely affected by the drug therapy, although folate deficiency did occur.

More information is becoming available about the use of statins in pediatric patients. In a 1-year trial, Stein et al. (JAMA 1999;281:137–144) randomized 132 boys aged 10–17 years with heterozygous FH to lovastatin or placebo. Compared with placebo, lovastatin 10, 20, and 40 mg/day reduced LDL-C by 17%, 24%, and 27%, and no significant differences were seen in growth, nutritional, or hormonal status or in clinical adverse events. In a shorter-term (12-week) placebo-controlled, randomized trial of pravastatin 5–20 mg/day in 72 children aged 8–16 years, Knipscheer et al. (Pediatr Res 1996;39[suppl 5]:867–871) demonstrated 23–32% reductions in LDL-C, with no safety concerns.

Table 3-1. Absolute Risk Estimates for ILIB Primary-Prevention Adult Cases According to PROCAM and Framingham Risk Calculators

Factor Included			ILIB Case								
PRO	Fram	Factor	1	2	3	4	5	6	7	8	13
40–65	30–74	Age	33	45	58	40	45	55	74	40	45
M/F	M/F	Sex	M	M	M	F	F	F	M	F	F
Y/N	Y/N	Smoker	N	Y	N	N	N	N	N	N	Y
	<160–280+	TC	258	191	240	215	293	219	250	500	336
25–75	<35–60+	HDL-C	60	31	30	39	85	41	40	—	48
50–400		TG	140	160	283	290	142	110	90	1,200	390
75–250	<100–190+	LDL-C	170	128	153	118	180	156	192	—	210
100–225	<120–160+	SBP	110	120	128	110	105	120	130	100	110
	<80–100+	DBP	70	80	84	70	70	80	80	70	70
Y/N	Y/N	DM	N	N	N	Y	N	N	N	N	N
Y/N	Y/N	Fam Hx MI	N	N	N	Y	N	Y	N	N	Y
		Other considerations		BMI 30.4, waist 96.5	BMI 28.0, waist 98, IGT, Hx hypertension	BMI 26.3, fam Hx type 2 DM	Hx hypertension	Sedentary	Hx hypertension; fam Hx stroke, CABG	BMI 41.0, waist 112, IGT	
PROCAM 8-yr risk (%)			2	3.7	10.4	1.3		5.2			10
Framingham 10-yr risk (%)			2	10	16	4	2	10	31	4	5
Av. same age & sex Framingham (%)			3	11	16	2	5	12	30	2	5

Note: Lipid values are mg/dL; blood pressure values are mm Hg; BMI values are kg/m²; waist circumference values are cm. DM = diabetes mellitus; IGT = impaired glucose tolerance.

Note: The percentage differences in risk estimates between PROCAM (Münster Heart Study) and Framingham may be largely explained by the different coronary endpoints used. Both calculators provide estimates for "hard" CHD, in PROCAM defined as fatal or nonfatal MI or sudden cardiac death and in Framingham defined as recognized or unrecognized MI (the latter defined by ECG), coronary insufficiency (unstable angina), or CHD death. Thus, PROCAM estimates probably accord well with combined endpoints in several clinical trials whereas Framingham estimates are somewhat higher although probably correspond closely to AFCAPS/TexCAPS endpoints (see 1.5.1). Definitions of CHD endpoints are critically important when risk cutpoints are defined to select patients for specific therapeutic interventions. For a full discussion of the appropriate use of multiple risk factor assessment equations, see Grundy et al. *J Am Coll Cardiol* 1999;34:1348–1359 (simultaneously published *Circulation* 1999;100:1481–1492).

A risk estimate has not been provided when any value is out of range. Although PROCAM 8-year risk was derived from men aged 40–65, it may be possible to extrapolate the estimates to postmenopausal women. The interactive PROCAM risk calculator is available at www.chd-taskforce.com. The Framingham risk charts (Wilson et al. *Circulation* 1998;97:1837–1847) are available on line at www.nhlbi.nih.gov/about/framingham/riskabs.htm; preliminary access to the charts in interactive form is at www.usnews.com/usnews/nycu/health/sfheart.htm.

APPENDIXES

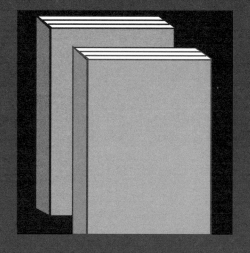

A. SOURCES: MAJOR ADULT CLINICAL RECOMMENDATIONS

A.1 Guidelines of the Second Adult Treatment Panel of the U.S. National Cholesterol Education Program

Table A.1-1. NCEP Lipid Screening in Adults

Age*	≥20 years
Appropriate screening	Universal, opportunistic
Measure nonfasting TC and HDL-C	• Healthy individuals
	• Proceed to fasting lipoprotein analysis if patient without atherosclerotic disease has high TC, low HDL-C, or borderline-high TC + ≥2 other risk factors (see Tables A.1-2 and A.1-3).
Perform full fasting lipoprotein analysis: TC, HDL-C, TG, and LDL-C	• Atherosclerotic disease present or
	• Diabetes mellitus present[†]
	• Advisable if patient otherwise at high risk (e.g., hypertension, family history of early CVD, multiple risk factors)
	• Physician may choose as the initial assessment in healthy individuals

Source: Data from Expert Panel on Detection, Evaluation, and Treatment of High Blood Cholesterol in Adults. Summary of the second report of the National Cholesterol Education Program (NCEP) Expert Panel on Detection, Evaluation, and Treatment of High Blood Cholesterol in Adults (Adult Treatment Panel II). *JAMA* 1993;269:3015–3023.

* For NCEP screening recommendations in children and adolescents, see Table B.2-1.

† The ADA recommends that a full fasting lipoprotein profile be obtained every year in adult patients with diabetes (see Appendix B.1).

Table A.1-2. NCEP Clinical Action According to Initial Cholesterol Values in Adults

Initial Assessment	Results and Action
Secondary prevention	
Fasting lipoprotein analysis*	LDL-C ≤100 (≤2.6): Individualized instruction on Step II Diet (see Table A.1-7) and other lifestyle modifications; repeat lipoprotein analysis annually
	LDL-C >100 (>2.6): Clinical evaluation; initiate cholesterol-lowering therapy
Primary prevention	
TC and HDL-C (nonfasting acceptable)	TC <200 (<5.2) HDL-C ≥35 (≥0.9): Repeat TC and HDL-C within 5 years or with physical examination; general educational materials
	HDL-C <35 (<0.9): Lipoprotein analysis (see below)
	TC 200–239 (5.2–6.1) HDL-C ≥35 (≥0.9) + <2 other RF: Repeat TC and HDL-C in 1–2 years; instruct in diet, physical activity, RF reduction
	HDL-C <35 (<0.9) or ≥2 other RF: Lipoprotein analysis (see below)
	TC ≥240 (≥6.2): Lipoprotein analysis (see below)
Fasting lipoprotein analysis†	LDL-C <130 (<3.4): Repeat TC and HDL-C within 5 years; general educational materials
	LDL-C 130–159 (3.4–4.0) <2 other RF: Information on Step I Diet (see Table A.1-7) and other lifestyle modifications. Reevaluate annually, including lipoprotein analysis, RF reduction
	≥2 other RF: Clinical evaluation; initiate dietary and other lifestyle modifications
	LDL-C ≥160 (≥4.1): Clinical evaluation; initiate dietary and other lifestyle modifications

Source: Data from Expert Panel on Detection, Evaluation, and Treatment of High Blood Cholesterol in Adults. Summary of the second report of the National Cholesterol Education Program (NCEP) Expert Panel on Detection, Evaluation, and Treatment of High Blood Cholesterol in Adults (Adult Treatment Panel II). *JAMA* 1993;269:3015–3023.

Note: RF = risk factor(s). Other risk factors for consideration in the NCEP algorithm are listed in Table A.1-3.

Note: All lipid values are mg/dL (mmol/L).

*Average of 2 determinations 1–8 wk apart (3 if variation >30 mg/dL, or >0.8 mmol/L); patient should not be in recovery phase from acute coronary or other medical event.

†May also be performed at outset. Assignment to last 2 categories (high risk) should be based on average of at least 2 determinations, as in previous footnote.

Table A.1-3. Other Major Risk Factors Considered in the Adult NCEP Algorithm

Risk Factor	Value/Comment
Positive*	
Age	Men ≥45 years Women ≥55 years, or premature menopause without ERT
Family history of premature CHD	Definite MI or sudden CHD death before age 55 years in male first-degree relative, or before age 65 years in female first-degree relative
Current cigarette smoking	No level of cigarette smoking is acceptable
Hypertension	Blood pressure ≥140/90 mm Hg or taking antihypertension medication
Low HDL-C	<35 mg/dL (<0.9 mmol/L)
Diabetes mellitus	Taking diabetic agent(s) or meets criteria for diagnosis (see Table B.1-1)
Obesity, in particular abdominal obesity[†]	(See Tables D.3-1 and D.3-2)
Negative (protective)	
High HDL-C	≥60 mg/dL (≥1.6): in adult primary-prevention algorithm, may subtract 1 risk factor other than hypercholesterolemia when high HDL-C is present

Source: Data modified from Expert Panel on Detection, Evaluation, and Treatment of High Blood Cholesterol in Adults. Summary of the second report of the National Cholesterol Education Program (NCEP) Expert Panel on Detection, Evaluation, and Treatment of High Blood Cholesterol in Adults (Adult Treatment Panel II). *JAMA* 1993;269:3015–3023.

Note: All lipid values are mg/dL (mmol/L).

Note: These are major risk factors for consideration in addition to elevated LDL-C and the presence of CHD or other atherosclerotic disease.

*Physical inactivity should also be a target for intervention.

†Obesity was not listed by the NCEP because its risk was considered to be accounted for by other factors (hypertension, hyperlipidemia, low HDL-C, and diabetes mellitus). It is listed here because the American Heart Association has since deemed obesity a major risk factor for CHD.

Table A.1-4. NCEP Action Limits for Consideration of Drug Therapy According to LDL-C Concentration in Adults

Patient Group	Initiation	Goal	Notes
No CHD, <2 other risk factors	≥190 (≥4.9)	<160 (<4.1)	• When LDL-C is 190–220 (4.9–5.7) and there is *no other risk,* consider delaying drug therapy in both men <35 years old and premenopausal women. • Use clinical judgment as to whether to use drugs after maximum lifestyle intervention when LDL-C is between 160 and 190 (4.1–4.9).
No CHD, ≥2 other risk factors	≥160 (≥4.1)	<130 (<3.4)	• Use clinical judgment as to whether to use drugs after maximum lifestyle intervention when LDL-C is between 130 and 160 (3.4–4.1).
With CHD or other atherosclerotic disease	≥130 (≥3.4)	≤100 (≤2.6)	An American Heart Association panel* has since recommended that: • Withholding drug therapy in an effort to reach target LDL-C with lifestyle changes is not necessary for LDL-C ≥130 (≥3.4). • A 6-week trial of lifestyle therapy is recommended when LDL-C is between 100 and 130 (2.6–3.4).

Source: Data from Expert Panel on Detection, Evaluation, and Treatment of High Blood Cholesterol in Adults. Summary of the second report of the National Cholesterol Education Program (NCEP) Expert Panel on Detection, Evaluation, and Treatment of High Blood Cholesterol in Adults (Adult Treatment Panel II). *JAMA* 1993;269:3015–3023.

Note: All lipid values are mg/dL (mmol/L).

Note: Additional risk factors to consider are listed in Table A.1-3.

*Grundy et al. *Circulation* 1997;95:2329–2331.

Table A.1-5. NCEP Recommendations for Management of HTG in Adults

Value	Category	Primary Management	Consideration of Drug Therapy
<200 (<2.3)	Acceptable		
200–400 (2.3–4.5)	Borderline high	• Control underlying conditions (see 2.5) • Control body weight • Institute diet* • Institute regular exercise • Restrict alcohol in selected patients • Stop smoking, for CVD health	• Established atherosclerotic disease • Family history of premature CHD • Concomitant TC ≥240 (≥6.2) and HDL-C <35 (<0.9) • Genetic form of dyslipidemia associated with increased CHD risk (e.g., FCH, familial type III hyperlipidemia) • In some cases, multiple risk factors • ADA leaves to clinical judgment in diabetes mellitus (see B.1.4.2)
400–1,000 (4.5–11.3)	High	• As above, with emphasis on controlling causes of 2° HTG • Values labile: can easily become very high	• Definitely use if history of acute pancreatitis • ADA advises strong consideration in diabetes mellitus (see B.1.4.2) • See also above
≥1,000 (≥11.3)	Very high	• Immediate, vigorous TG-lowering efforts required because of risk for acute pancreatitis • Drugs are effective to lower VLDL (see Table 2.9-3), but no available drug is effective in lowering chylomicron concentrations • Treat causes of 2° HTG, including discontinuation of drugs that raise TG (see Table 2.5-1) • Very low fat diet; avoid alcohol†	

Source: Data from National Cholesterol Education Program. Second report of the Expert Panel on Detection, Evaluation, and Treatment of High Blood Cholesterol in Adults (Adult Treatment Panel II). *Circulation* 1994;89:1329–1445.

Note: All lipid values are mg/dL (mmol/L).

Note: Goal is to reduce TG to <200 (<2.3). Some authorities, including the ILIB, consider TG <150 (<1.7) desirable.

*Increasing the ratio of monounsaturated to saturated fatty acids and increasing the proportion of carbohydrate calories obtained from complex carbohydrates are important aspects of the lipid-lowering diet in patients with HTG.

†In type I hyperlipidemia, use diet with <10% of total energy intake as fat and with low intake of simple carbohydrates; alcohol avoidance; and weight control. Substitution of medium-chain for long-chain fatty acids may be helpful in type I.

Table A.1-6. NCEP Recommendations for Increasing Low HDL-C in Adults

Value	Category	Primary Management	Consideration of Drug Therapy
<35 mg/dL (<0.9 mmol/L)	Low (high-risk) HDL-C	• Control body weight • Stop smoking • Institute regular exercise • Address concurrent agents that lower HDL-C (see 2.5)	• Consider HDL-C value in selection of drug(s) to lower LDL-C • Use not recommended for isolated low HDL-C in low-risk primary prevention

Source: Data from National Cholesterol Education Program. Second report of the Expert Panel on Detection, Evaluation, and Treatment of High Blood Cholesterol in Adults (Adult Treatment Panel II). *Circulation* 1994;89:1329–1445.

Table A.1-7. Step I and II Diets of the NCEP and American Heart Association

	Recommended Intake	
Nutrient*	Step I Diet (Primary Prevention)	Step II Diet (Primary or Secondary Prevention[†])
Total fat[‡]	≤30% of total calories	
Saturated fatty acids	8–10% of total calories	<7% of total calories
Polyunsaturated fatty acids	≤10% of total calories	
Monounsaturated fatty acids	≤15% of total calories	
Carbohydrates	≥55% of total calories	
Protein	~15% of total calories	
Cholesterol	<300 mg/day	<200 mg/day
Total calories	Adults: To achieve and maintain desirable weight. Children and adolescents: To promote normal growth and development and to reach or maintain desirable weight	

Source: Data from Expert Panel on Detection, Evaluation, and Treatment of High Blood Cholesterol in Adults. Summary of the second report of the National Cholesterol Education Program (NCEP) Expert Panel on Detection, Evaluation, and Treatment of High Blood Cholesterol in Adults (Adult Treatment Panel II). JAMA 1993;269:3015–3023.

Note: For cardiovascular health, it is also advisable to limit sodium intake to <2,400 mg/day and to limit alcohol intake to moderate levels.

*Calories from alcohol not included.

†The Step II Diet is initial dietary intervention in patients with atherosclerotic disease; it may be initial dietary intervention in primary prevention if the patient has already been complying with a diet equivalent to the Step I Diet.

‡It is also advisable to limit intake of foods high in trans fatty acids.

A.2 Recommendations of the Second Joint Task Force of European and Other Societies on Coronary Prevention

Table A.2-1. Joint Task Force Lifestyle and Therapeutic Goals for Adults with CHD or Other Atherosclerotic Disease and for High-Risk Healthy Individuals

Patients with CHD or Other Atherosclerotic Disease	High-Risk Healthy Individuals*
Lifestyle	
Stop smoking, make healthy food choices, be physically active, and achieve ideal weight.	
Other risk factors	
Blood pressure <140/90 mm Hg TC <190 mg/dL (<5.0 mmol/L) LDL-C <115 mg/dL (<3.0 mmol/L) When these risk factor goals are not achieved by lifestyle changes, blood pressure and cholesterol-lowering drug therapies should be used.	
Other prophylactic drug therapies	
Aspirin (at least 75 mg) for all coronary patients and those with cerebral atherosclerosis or PVD	Aspirin (75 mg) in treated hypertensive patients
Beta-blockers in post-MI patients	
ACE inhibitors in patients with symptoms or signs of heart failure at the time of MI or with chronic LV systolic dysfunction (ejection fraction <40%)	
Anticoagulants in selected coronary patients	
Screen close relatives	
Of patients with premature CHD (men <55 years, women <65 years)	If FH or other inherited dyslipidemia is suspected

Source: Prevention of coronary heart disease in clinical practice. Recommendations of the Second Joint Task Force of European and other Societies on Coronary Prevention. *Eur Heart J* 1998;19:1434–1503; used with permission. The full recommendations are also available at www.escardio.org (see "Guidelines and Scientific Statements" in "Scientific and Clinical Information").

*Absolute risk for CHD ≥20% over 10 years or will exceed 20% if projected to age 60.

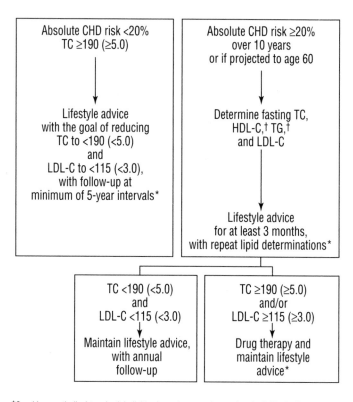

*Consider genetically determined dyslipidemias and causes of secondary dyslipidemia. If appropriate, refer to a specialist.

†HDL-C <40 (<1.0) and fasting TG >180 (>2.0) are markers of increased coronary risk.

Figure A.2-1. Lipid management for primary prevention of CHD in adults—Joint Task Force recommendations. All lipid values are mg/dL (mmol/L). The Joint Task Force provides in its guidelines a risk chart encompassing sex, age, smoking status, TC, and SBP for estimating 10-year absolute risk for a CHD event (angina, nonfatal MI, or coronary death) in individuals who do not have known atherosclerotic disease. Modified in format from Prevention of coronary heart disease in clinical practice. Recommendations of the Second Joint Task Force of European and other Societies on Coronary Prevention. *Eur Heart J* 1998;19:1434–1503; used with permission. Recommendations also available at www.escardio.org.

B. POPULATION SUBSETS

B.1 Management of Dyslipidemia in Adults with Diabetes Mellitus

B.1.1 Diagnosis and Classification of Diabetes

The diagnostic criteria of the American Diabetes Association (ADA) for diabetes mellitus were revised in 1997 (Expert Committee *Diabetes Care* 1997;20:1183–1197). The new criteria are shown in Table B.1-1. The key change is lowering of the fasting plasma glucose cutpoint for diagnosis of diabetes. The venous fasting plasma glucose concentration is considered normal when it is <110 mg/dL (<6.1 mmol/L). Fasting plasma glucose values of 110–125 mg/dL (6.1–6.9 mmol/L) define impaired fasting glucose tolerance. Diabetes is diagnosed when the fasting glucose value is ≥126 mg/dL (≥7.0 mmol/L). By the old criteria, a fasting glucose value ≥140 mg/dL, or ≥7.8 mmol/L, indicated diabetes. As with the previous criteria, impaired glucose tolerance is defined by 2-hour plasma glucose values 140–200 mg/dL (7.8–11.1 mmol/L) during an oral glucose tolerance test using 75 g glucose dissolved in water. Impaired glucose tolerance is not a disease entity, but individuals in this category are at increased risk for CVD, microvascular complications, and diabetes.

The classification of diabetes was revised as well. The terms *insulin-dependent diabetes mellitus* (IDDM) and *non-insulin-dependent diabetes mellitus* (NIDDM) were eliminated; the terms *type 1* and *type 2 diabetes mellitus* are retained. Patients with type 1 diabetes are prone to ketoacidosis; most cases of type 1 are due to pancreatic islet beta cell destruction (usually by autoimmune processes). Type 2 diabetes, which accounts for >90% of cases of diabetes mellitus, results from insulin resistance with an insulin secretory defect. Obesity, which is prevalent in type 2, further contributes to the insulin resistance. The hyperglycemia develops gradually, and type 2 diabetes frequently goes undiagnosed for many years: individuals with even severe hyperglycemia can remain largely asymptomatic for long periods. Epidemiologic studies in the United States have shown that 50% of individuals with diabetes are undiagnosed (Harris et al. *Diabetes* 1987;36:523–534). At diagnosis, 20% of patients with type 2 diabetes have retinopathy, 9% have neuropathy, 8% have nephropathy, and the prevalence of macrovascular complications is similar to that in patients with diabetes not newly diagnosed (Engelgau et al. *Diabetes Care* 1995;18:1606–1618). Risk is markedly increased for microvascular and macrovascular complications in both types 1 and 2.

Diabetes is estimated to affect at least 100 million people worldwide, and a worldwide increase (which translates into a significant economic impact) is expected as people in industrialized societies age and as lifestyles in industrializing nations become westernized. The primary prevention of type 2 diabetes—in chief through weight control and exercise—is an urgent priority.

B.1.2 Atherosclerotic Disease in Diabetes

Seventy-five to eighty percent of adults with diabetes mellitus die of atherosclerotic disease; CHD accounts for three fourths of those deaths, cerebrovascular and PVD events for the remainder. In most studies, the excess risks for CHD and PVD are relatively greater in diabetic women than in diabetic men.

Type 2 diabetes increases CHD risk two to three times in men and three to seven times in women; it nearly eliminates any female premenopausal cardioprotection. Concomitant risk factors such as dyslipidemia, hypertension, and abdominal obesity are common in adults with type 2 diabetes; however, the contribution of diabetes to CHD risk appears to be in part independent of such associated factors. Possible direct deleterious effects of insulin include mitogenic properties and inhibition of endogenous fibrinolysis. Decreased fibrinolytic activity, increased procoagulant activity, decreased anticoagulant activity, and increased platelet aggregation described in diabetes are likely to predispose to atherothrombosis. The risk factor clustering in type 2 diabetes may represent a genetic interlinkage (see the description of the cardiovascular metabolic syndrome in 1.3.6).

At 12-year follow-up of **Multiple Risk Factor Intervention Trial** (MRFIT) screenees, absolute risk for CVD mortality was much higher for the diabetic than the nondiabetic men at every age and risk factor level, and risk increased more steeply in the diabetic men as risk factor levels rose (Stamler et al. *Diabetes Care* 1993;16:434–444). At 7-year follow-up of 2,432 subjects who were part of a well-characterized Finnish population-based cohort, adjusted risk for CHD death was not significantly different between diabetic subjects without previous MI and nondiabetic subjects with a history of MI (Haffner et al. *N Engl J Med* 1998;339:229–234). In diabetic patients the mortality rate (including the prehospital mortality rate) after MI is high, as are complication and failure rates after interventions such as CABG and PTCA.

Because of the high CVD risk, it is particularly important to achieve risk factor goals in diabetic patients, and more stringent goals for some factors appear to be appropriate. The absolute benefit of reducing risk factors in diabetic patients is likely to be greater than like intervention in nondiabetic patients. The multiple risk factor approach includes medical nutrition therapy, weight reduction when indicated, increased physical activity, and the use of oral glucose-lowering agents and/or insulin, with careful attention to other CVD risk factors (Table B.1-2). Intervention must be vigorous. Lifestyle changes to reduce risk for macrovascular disease will also likely help prevent progression of insulin resistance and diabetes.

Evidence supports increased risk for macrovascular disease at even slight elevations of fasting plasma glucose. Regardless of the HbA_{1c} value, fasting glucose >110 mg/dL (>6.1 mmol/L) (and perhaps even >90 mg/dL, or >5.0 mmol/L) confers high risk for macrovascular disease. It is estimated that 63% of patients with fasting plasma glucose ≥126 mg/dL will have a normal HbA_{1c} value (4.3–6.3%), and only 7% will have a value >7% (Peters et al. *JAMA* 1996;276:1246–1252; Peters *Prev Cardiol* 1998;Spring:57–59). But while the patients with normal HbA_{1c} are probably at fairly low risk for microvascular complications, their glucose tolerance is not normal. They have significant insulin resistance, and their risk for macrovascular disease is very high. Management of their CHD risk factors must be aggressive, and they should be monitored for worsening of glycemic status.

The **Diabetes Control and Complications Trial** (DCCT) in type 1 disease and the **United Kingdom Prospective Diabetes Study** (UKPDS) in type 2 disease convincingly demonstrated the protective value of tight blood glucose control in preventing microvascular complications of diabetes. However, neither study unequivocally demonstrated that intensive glucose control has benefit for macrovascular disease events. In DCCT ($N = 1,441$), cardiac and PVD events were reduced 41% (p = 0.06) in the intensive insulin therapy group (median HbA_{1c} achieved 7.2%, vs. 9.1% in the conventional therapy group) (The Diabetes Control and Complications Trial Research Group *N Engl J Med* 1993;329:977–986). At diagnosis of diabetes in UKPDS (median age 53 years), 50% of subjects already had signs of diabetic tissue damage; 8% had CVD. The multifactorial nature of the CVD assessed in UKPDS probably made it unlikely that a clear answer would emerge, and the stepwise use of glucose-lowering agents has made interpretation of the effects of individual agents difficult. In the UKPDS test of intensive therapy with sulfonylureas or insulin versus conventional therapy (N = 3,867; median HbA_{1c} achieved 7.0% vs. 7.9%), intensive therapy achieved a borderline decrease in MI rate (p = 0.052) but no difference in PVD. There was a greater increase in weight as well as increased risk for hypoglycemic episodes with this intensive therapy compared with conventional therapy (UK Prospective Diabetes Study Group *Lancet* 1998;352:837–853). In overweight patients in UKPDS (>120% ideal body weight), metformin versus conventional therapy (N = 1,704; median HbA_{1c} achieved 7.4% vs. 8.0%) significantly reduced risk for any diabetes-related endpoint, for diabetes-related death, and for all-cause mortality. Early addition of metformin in sulfonylurea-treated overweight patients, however, significantly increased risk for diabetes-related death (UK Prospective Diabetes Study Group *Lancet* 1998;352:854–865). That finding merits close attention but might be interpreted to reflect a progressive loss of beta-cell function. Metformin therapy was associated with less weight gain and fewer hypoglycemic episodes than were sulfonylureas or insulin. Aggressive control of hypertension in the UKPDS patients, with a beta-blocker or an ACE inhibitor as the main treatment, reduced both macrovascular and microvascular event rates (UK Prospective Diabetes Study Group *BMJ* 1998;317:703–713, 713–720). A nonsignificant 54% reduction in cardiovascular complications, together with significantly reduced microvascular complications, was achieved with intensive insulin therapy in the small **Kumamoto Study** (N = 110), also conducted in type 2 diabetes (Ohkubo et al. *Diabetes Res Clin Pract* 1995;28:103–117).

B.1.3 Dyslipidemia in Diabetes

The most common lipid abnormalities in diabetes, particularly type 2 diabetes, are increased plasma TG and decreased HDL-C. Considerable evidence indicates that these abnormalities may be intrinsically related to the abnormal physiology produced by insulin resistance or inadequate insulin action. Familial lipid disorders such as FCH and familial HTG, which occur often in subjects with type 2 diabetes, may contribute to the severe TG elevations seen in some patients with diabetes, as may hypothyroidism, renal disease, and use of alcohol or estrogens. In many studies, dyslipidemia is more severe in diabetic women than in diabetic men, consistent with the relatively greater risk for atherosclerotic disease events in diabetic women.

Elevated LDL-C may also be present in diabetes. Typically, LDL-C values are not different from those in nondiabetic subjects. However, subjects with type 2 diabetes tend to have small, dense LDL, which may be associated with the described cardiovascular metabolic syndrome (see 1.3.6), and there is evidence that LDL from diabetic subjects is more susceptible to nonenzymatic glycosylation (which may slow its clearance from plasma, among other possible consequences) and oxidative modification. (See also B.1.5 below.)

B.1.3.1 Data from Clinical Trials of Lipid-Regulating Drugs

No reported large pharmacologic lipid-regulating trial has been restricted to diabetic patients. Subset analyses are available, however, from major trials, including the **Scandinavian Simvastatin Survival Study** (4S) (Pyörälä et al. *Diabetes Care* 1997;20:614–620), **Cholesterol and Recurrent Events** (CARE) trial (Goldberg et al. *Circulation* 1998;98:2513–2519), **Long-term Intervention with Pravastatin in Ischemic Disease** (LIPID) trial (LIPID Study Group *N Engl J Med* 1998;339:1349–1357), and **Veterans Affairs Cooperative Studies Program High-Density Lipoprotein Cholesterol Intervention Trial** (HIT) (Rubins et al. *N Engl J Med* 1999;341:410–418) in patients with CHD, as well as the **Helsinki Heart Study** (Koskinen et al. *Diabetes Care* 1992;15:820–825) in primary prevention. As seen in Table B.1-3, subjects with diabetes accounted for fairly small percentages of enrollees in the trials, and CHD risk reduction was similar between diabetic and nondiabetic patients. In 4S the all-cause mortality rate was also reduced, by 43% (compared with 28% in nondiabetic patients), as was risk for cerebrovascular events (-62%). In CARE, the statistically significant reductions in all-cause stroke (-32%) and stroke or TIA (-27%) were independent of potential covariates, including diabetes (Plehn et al. *Circulation* 1999;99:216–223). The recurrent coronary event rate also tended to be lower among glucose-intolerant patients in CARE. In the LIPID substudy examining carotid lesion progression by B-mode ultrasound, 5% of the subjects were diabetic. Their results were consonant with findings in nondiabetic subjects, namely, treatment's prevention of any detectable increase in carotid wall thickening over 4 years of follow-up (MacMahon et al. *Circulation* 1998;97:1784–1790). Angiographic benefit of aggressive cholesterol-lowering therapy with lovastatin (and cholestyramine as necessary) in the **Post Coronary Artery Bypass** (Post-CABG) trial was similar between diabetic and nondiabetic subjects (Hoogwerf et al. *Diabetes* 1999;48:1289–1294). The diabetic patients in 4S, CARE, and the Helsinki Heart Study were older, more obese, and more likely to be hypertensive than their nondiabetic counterparts (LIPID and HIT diabetes results have not yet been separately reported), and diabetic patients in the placebo groups were 1.5–2 times more likely to have a coronary event than nondiabetic placebo recipients.

Although the reduction in coronary events in diabetic subjects in LIPID was not statistically significant, perhaps because of underpowering, the investigators saw no evidence of significant heterogeneity of treatment effect among predefined subgroups, including diabetic subjects. The Helsinki investigators advised caution in interpretation of the 60% CHD risk reduction in their trial because of the small numbers of diabetic subjects and events. Still, **absolute benefits of treatment are likely to be greater among individuals at higher absolute risk.** In 4S, absolute risk reduction was 8.1% in diabetic patients, compared with 5.2% in nondiabetic patients. The probability of escaping a major CHD event in 4S was 51% in diabetic placebo recipients, 75% in diabetic patients randomized to simvastatin, 71% in nondiabetic placebo recipients, and 80% in nondiabetic patients randomized to simvastatin.

The small ($N = 164$), double-blind **St. Mary's, Ealing, Northwick Park Diabetes Cardiovascular Disease Prevention** (SENDCAP) study, restricted to patients with type 2 diabetes and no clinical evidence of CVD, also yielded suggestive results. Patients were randomized to receive bezafibrate or placebo for 3 years, bezafibrate therapy yielding a TG reduction of 32%, HDL-C increase of 6%, and TC reduction of 7%, compared with baseline values of 198, 39, and 223 mg/dL (or 2.2, 1.0, and 5.8 mmol/L). Although there was no significant difference between the groups in carotid progression (the primary endpoint) as measured by B-mode ultrasound, the rate of CHD events (a secondary endpoint, defined as probable ischemic change on resting ECG plus documented MI) was significantly reduced (p = 0.01) in the bezafibrate group (Elkeles et al. *Diabetes Care* 1998;21:641–648).

(See 1.5 and 1.6 for a general discussion of cholesterol-lowering trials.)

B.1.4 ADA Recommendations

ADA practice guidelines now include the management of dyslipidemia (ADA *Diabetes Care* 1999;22:S56–S59). The ILIB endorses the recommendations of the ADA, with the noted additions. Because of the data from trials of LDL-C lowering, the ADA places primary emphasis on intervention against LDL-C. It notes, however, that raising low HDL-C and reducing elevated TG may also be useful, and those dyslipidemias are targets for intervention.

A full fasting lipoprotein profile should be obtained every year in adult patients with diabetes, in particular because changes in glycemic control affect lipoproteins. Assessment may be decreased to once every 2 years if lipid values are low risk. As in the general population, it is usually recommended that at least two fasting blood samples be taken at least 1 week apart before a treatment decision regarding dyslipidemia is finalized. Patients with TG exceeding 1,000 mg/dL (11.3 mmol/L) are at high risk for acute pancreatitis and need special, immediate attention, including pharmacotherapy and severe dietary fat restriction. In the presence of elevated LDL-C, serum thyroid-stimulating hormone should be tested to rule out hypothyroidism, a not uncommon clinical finding in type 2 diabetes. Both hypothyroidism and type 2 diabetes are common disorders in the elderly.

Because of the high risk for CHD, the ADA considers an LDL-C value ≤100 mg/dL (≤2.6 mmol/L) optimal in all adult patients with type 2 diabetes, that is, the target recommended in the NCEP guidelines for patients with CHD. Action limits for LDL-C reduction are shown in Table B.1-4. ADA definitions of higher, borderline, and lower risk levels according to HDL-C and fasting TG concentrations are shown in Table B.1-5; as noted there, the

ILIB considers lower cutpoints for risk according to fasting TG desirable. Priorities for treatment of diabetic dyslipidemia are shown in Table B.1-6. The ILIB notes that particular emphasis should be placed on determining whether macrovascular disease is present. The ILIB algorithm shown in Chart B.1-1 (page 134) derives from the LDL-C and HDL-C management recommendations of the 1999 ADA practice guidelines and the TG management recommendations of the 1993 ADA consensus panel (*Diabetes Care* 1993;16[suppl 2]:106–112).

B.1.4.1 Treatment of Dyslipidemia by Lifestyle Changes and Glycemic Control

Reduction of overweight, a low-fat diet, regular physical activity, and glycemic control are fundamental to lipid management in the diabetic population. The approach to weight control should be aggressive. Alcohol reduction or abstention is advisable when HTG is present.

Control of hyperglycemia may greatly improve abnormal lipid values, particularly in type 1 diabetes. Effects on TG tend to be greatest, and usually reflect the degree of glycemic control. Effects on HDL-C are more variable, and LDL-C may decrease modestly. HDL composition may be altered in a direction believed to be antiatherogenic, as may LDL composition when plasma TG decreases. Previous debates about the lipid effects of particular diabetic agents may be of reduced relevance because multiagent therapy is now common. Metformin has consistently been shown to improve lipid values, including not only TG lowering but also apparently LDL-C lowering and possibly HDL-C raising, all the changes modest. Metformin's effects on the fibrinolytic system would be expected to enhance fibrinolysis. Improved glycemic control with insulin possibly has a greater effect on HDL-C than improved glycemic control with sulfonylureas.

B.1.4.2 Lipid-Regulating Drug Therapy

As in the treatment of any dyslipidemic patient, lipid-regulating pharmacotherapy supplements rather than replaces nonpharmacologic measures. The ADA recommends that lifestyle and lipid-regulating drug therapies begin simultaneously in diabetic patients when clinical atherosclerotic disease is present or in primary prevention when LDL-C is very high ($\geq$200 mg/dL, or $\geq$5.2 mmol/L). Also, when averaged LDL-C at the beginning of therapy in a diabetic patient without atherosclerosis exceeds the LDL-C goal (Table B.1-4) by >25 mg/dL (>0.6 mmol/L), the physician may choose to begin lipid-regulating pharmacotherapy at the same time as behavioral therapy in patients at high risk, including some patients with multiple risk factors. Otherwise, effectiveness of behavioral interventions may be evaluated every 6 weeks, with consideration of lipid-regulating drug therapy at 3–6 months. Changes in pharmacotherapy should be made at intervals of about 4 to 6 weeks on the basis of laboratory findings.

Pharmacologically increasing HDL-C in diabetic patients is difficult because nicotinic acid, the most effective agent for increasing HDL-C, has a relative contraindication in the disease. Weight loss, smoking cessation, and increased physical activity may increase HDL-C.

When glycemic control has been improved as much as is likely, addition of a fibrate to reduce elevated plasma TG may be considered. The ADA advises that strong consideration should be given to pharmacotherapy when TG remains >400 mg/dL (>4.5 mmol/L); physicians are referred to clinical judgment for values of 200–400 mg/dL (2.3–4.5 mmol/L). The ILIB supports more aggressive TG-lowering efforts. In agreement with the 1993 consensus panel, it recommends consideration of TG-lowering drug therapy when TG remains >150 mg/dL (>1.7 mmol/L) despite lifestyle therapy and glycemic control in diabetic patients with atherosclerotic disease, or ≥400 mg/dL (≥4.5 mmol/L) in the absence of other risk factors or ≥200 mg/dL (≥2.3 mmol/L) in the presence of other risk factors in primary prevention. Drug choice considerations are outlined in Table B.1-6.

B.1.5 Considerations in Adults with Type 1 Diabetes

Risk for atherosclerotic disease in type 1 diabetes is almost equivalent to that of heterozygous familial hypercholesterolemia. Data from the Joslin Clinic showed that 35% of patients with type 1 diabetes died of CHD by age 55, compared with only 8% of nondiabetic men and 4% of nondiabetic women (Krolewski et al. *Am J Cardiol* 1987;59:750–755). In patients with type 1 diabetes without albuminuria who have good glycemic control, plasma lipid concentrations tend to be normal, and sometimes are even better than normal. HTG or even chylomicronemia may be seen in very poorly controlled type 1 diabetes. When LDL-C exceeds the goals recommended in type 2 diabetes, the ADA considers aggressive treatment in type 1 reasonable, although no clinical trial data and only limited observational epidemiologic findings are available regarding lipid concentrations and CHD risk in type 1 diabetes. Intensive insulin therapy may decrease elevated plasma LDL-C and in some cases is associated with increased HDL-C. In some patients with type 1 diabetes, lipoproteins are abnormal in composition (e.g., an increased ratio of cholesterol to TG in VLDL), although clinical significance has not been demonstrated. Such compositional abnormalities may not resolve with intensive glucose control by insulin.

Table B.1-1. ADA Criteria for the Diagnosis of Diabetes Mellitus

Symptoms of diabetes (polyuria, polydipsia, unexplained weight loss) plus casual plasma glucose concentration ≥200 mg/dL (≥11.1 mmol/L), casual defined as any time of the day without regard to time since last meal

OR

Fasting plasma glucose ≥126 mg/dL (≥7.0 mmol/L), fasting defined as no caloric intake for at least 8 hours

OR

Two-hour plasma glucose ≥200 mg/dL (≥11.1 mmol/L) during an oral glucose tolerance test using a glucose load containing the equivalent of 75 g anhydrous glucose dissolved in water

Source: The Expert Committee. Report of the Expert Committee on the Diagnosis and Classification of Diabetes Mellitus. *Diabetes Care* 1999;22(suppl 1):S5–S19; used with permission.

Table B.1-2. Risk Factor Control in Diabetes Mellitus

GLUCOSE CONTROL

Careful diabetic control is essential. Goal: glycosylated hemoglobin (HbA_{1c}) <7.0% (ADA)

Use diet, exercise, and, as needed, oral agents and/or insulin.

Sulfonylureas: Achieve acceptable glycemic control in many patients with type 2 diabetes. Proven efficacy, well-defined mechanism of action, low cost, well-defined adverse effects.

Metformin: Increases sensitivity to endogenous insulin (enhancing insulin-mediated glucose uptake in muscle) and reduces plasma glucose and insulin concentrations. Ineffective in the absence of insulin. Reduces lipolysis and free fatty acid concentrations and improves the lipid profile. In the absence of renal abnormalities, can be beneficial in glycemic and lipid control in type 2 diabetes.

Insulin secretagogues: Repaglinide and nateglinide are new drugs that stimulate insulin secretion in the presence of glucose, as in the postprandial period. They are taken before meals and have demonstrated efficacy in reducing postprandial glycemic excursion in type 2 diabetes.

Insulin sensitizers: A new group of drugs, referred to also as thiazolidinediones (e.g., rosiglitazone, pioglitazone), that lower blood glucose concentrations by enhancing insulin action. This is achieved by increasing peripheral glucose disposal and decreasing hepatic glucose output through activation of peroxisome proliferator–activated receptor (PPAR) γ. Reductions in circulating concentrations of insulin, TG, and nonesterified fatty acids also occur. Insulin sensitizers act additively with other oral antidiabetic agents (sulfonylureas, metformin), and they reduce the insulin dosage required in insulin-treated patients. If dietary measures are not enforced, long-term treatment may lead to obesity. Troglitazone was withdrawn from the market because of hepatic toxicity. According to the U.S. Food and Drug Administration, data to date show that rosiglitazone and pioglitazone offer the same benefits as troglitazone without the same risks.

Alpha-glucosidase inhibitors: These agents (acarbose, miglitol) lower blood glucose by interfering with the intestinal digestion of CHO. Primary benefits are a reduction in postprandial glycemia and a decrease in the extremes between maximal and minimal postprandial glucose concentrations. The agents may be used in types 1 and 2 diabetes; their major drawback is flatulence and abdominal discomfort.

MEDICAL NUTRITION THERAPY

Individualize in all patients with diabetes, with referral to a dietitian for diet planning and appropriate nutrition education.

ADA dietary recommendations are similar to the general cholesterol-lowering diet (see 2.8), including reduced saturated fat and cholesterol, but include a higher-CHO diet or a higher-fat diet enriched in polyunsaturated or (if TG and VLDL are the primary concerns) monounsaturated fat. Omega-3 fatty acids provided naturally in seafood need not be curtailed. The ADA gives priority to CHO amount rather than type; other authorities emphasize complex CHO and restrict sugar. Weight loss may be difficult with a higher-fat diet.

Alcohol reduction or abstention is advisable when a concomitant medical condition such as HTG, pancreatitis, or neuropathy is present; otherwise, moderate alcohol intake (≤1 drink/day for women and lighter-weight men, otherwise ≤2 drinks/day) is permitted WITH FOOD in patients with good diabetic control. Restrict sodium to <2,400 mg/day in hypertensive patients.

CORRECTION OF OVERWEIGHT OR OBESITY

Weight control is essential to improved control of diabetes and associated CVD risk factors.

Special experience is required for intervention in insulin-treated patients.

Continued on next page

Table B.1-2—*Continued*

INCREASED PHYSICAL ACTIVITY

Increased physical activity improves insulin sensitivity in muscles, reduces plasma TG, and increases HDL-C.

Long-term programs of regular exercise are feasible for patients with uncomplicated type 2 diabetes.

Take into account that many diabetic patients have a low level of fitness. Precautions include thorough screening, precautions regarding the feet, careful warm-up and cool-down, proper hydration, avoidance of high-resistance exercise in older individuals and those with long-standing diabetes, and choice of appropriate exercise when there is loss of protective sensation.

SMOKING CESSATION

Goal: complete cessation mandatory. Young patients should be encouraged not to start smoking.

Smoking quadruples CHD risk in diabetic subjects. It increases their CVD risk up to 14 times (vs. smoking or diabetes alone); 95% of diabetic patients who require amputation are smokers.

The elimination of major metabolites of bupropion may be affected by reduced renal function.

CONTROL OF DYSLIPIDEMIA

Goals: LDL-C ≤100 mg/dL (≤2.6 mmol/L); HDL-C ≥35 mg/dL (≥0.9 mmol/L) in men and ≥45 mg/dL (≥1.2 mmol/L) in women, preferably >45 mg/dL (>1.2 mmol/L) in men and >55 (>1.4 mmol/L) in women; fasting TG <200 mg/dL (<2.3 mmol/L) (ADA). The ILIB recommends TG <150 mg/dL (<1.7 mmol/L) in diabetic patients and a minimal HDL-C goal of >45 mg/dL (>1.2 mmol/L) in all patients.

See accompanying text and tables.

CONTROL OF HYPERTENSION

Goal: blood pressure <130/85 mm Hg (ADA, JNC VI)

Measure blood pressure in the supine, sitting, and standing positions in all diabetic patients to detect evidence of autonomic dysfunction and orthostatic hypotension; automated ambulatory monitoring may be particularly helpful.

ACE inhibitors, alpha-blockers, calcium antagonists, and low-dosage diuretics have reduced adverse effects on glucose homeostasis, the lipid profile, and renal function; they are recommended as first-choice agents in diabetic patients by the JNC VI. However, diuretics and beta-blockers have yielded as much or more CVD risk reduction in diabetic as in nondiabetic patients; they are recommended as first-line agents by the International Task Force/International Atherosclerosis Society, with replacement if diabetic control or dyslipidemia worsens. The JNC VI recommends ACE inhibitors in patients with diabetic nephropathy; angiotensin II receptor blockers may be considered if ACE inhibitors are contraindicated or not well tolerated, and renoprotection has also been reported with use of a calcium antagonist.

MANAGEMENT OF DEPRESSION

Major depression, which is 3 times more common in diabetic adults than in the general adult population, adversely affects health behaviors necessary for good management of diabetes and is a health issue in itself.

Note: CHO = carbohydrate; JNC VI = U.S. Sixth Joint National Committee.

Note: Detailed intervention recommendations are available from the ADA at www.diabetes.org.

Table B.1-3. Findings in Diabetic Subjects in Clinical Endpoint Trials of Lipid-Regulating Drug Therapy

Trial (Agent)	N (%)	Mean Baseline LDL-C, HDL-C, TG in mg/dL (mmol/L)	% CHD Relative Risk Reduction with Drug Therapy (vs. Nondiabetic)	% CHD Events in Placebo Group (vs. Nondiabetic)
Secondary prevention				
4S (simvastatin)	202 (5)	187 (4.8), 44 (1.1), 152 (1.7)	55 (vs. 32)	45 (vs. 27)
CARE (pravastatin)	586 (14)	136 (3.5), 38 (1.0), 164 (1.9)	25 (vs. 23)	37 (vs. 25)
LIPID (pravastatin)	782 (9)	—	19 NS (vs. 25)	23 (vs. 15)
HIT (gemfibrozil)	627 (25)	—	24 (vs. 24)*	36 (vs. 23)
Primary prevention				
Helsinki (gemfibrozil)	135 (3)	200 (5.2), 46 (1.2), 239 (2.7)	60 NS (no data given for nondiabetic)	7.4 (vs. 3.3) for all patients

Note: See text for full names of trials.

*Relative risk reductions in combined secondary endpoint of CHD death, nonfatal MI, and confirmed stroke; p = 0.05 in diabetic patients.

Table B.1-4. Treatment Decisions Based on LDL-C in Adults with Type 2 Diabetes Mellitus— ADA Recommendations

	Medical Nutrition Therapy		Drug Therapy	
	Initiation	LDL-C Goal	Initiation*	LDL-C Goal
With known atherosclerotic disease	>100 (>2.6)	≤100 (≤2.6)	>100 (>2.6)	≤100 (≤2.6)
Without known atherosclerotic disease	>100 (>2.6)	≤100 (≤2.6)	≥130 (≥3.4)†	≤100 (≤2.6)

Source: American Diabetes Association. Management of dyslipidemia in adults with diabetes (position statement). *Diabetes Care* 1999;22(suppl 1):S56–S59; used with permission.

Note: All lipid values are mg/dL (mmol/L).

*In general in primary prevention, behavioral interventions should be tried for 3–6 months before lipid-regulating drug therapy is considered. Behavioral and pharmacologic interventions should be initiated at the same time, however, when LDL-C is very high (≥200, or ≥5.2). In addition, simultaneous initiation in primary prevention may be considered when LDL-C is ≥125 (≥3.2) and other risk is present. In secondary prevention, behavioral and pharmacologic interventions should be instituted simultaneously when LDL-C exceeds 100 (2.6).

†For primary-prevention diabetic patients who have multiple CHD risk factors, some authorities recommend initiation of drug therapy when LDL-C exceeds 100 (2.6). Other risk factors to consider are HDL-C <35 (<0.9) in men or HDL-C <45 (<1.2) in women; hypertension; smoking; family history of premature CVD; or microalbuminuria or proteinuria. Age and sex are not considered risk factors because diabetic men and women are considered to have equal CVD risk.

Table B.1-5. Risk for Atherosclerotic Disease According to HDL-C and Fasting TG Concentrations— ADA Definitions

	HDL-C		TG
Risk	M	F	Both Sexes
Higher	<35 (<0.9)	<45 (<1.2)	≥400 (≥4.5)
Borderline	35–45 (0.9–1.2)	45–55 (1.2–1.4)	200–399 (2.3–4.5)
Lower	>45 (>1.2)	>55 (>1.4)	<200 (<2.3)

Source: Data from American Diabetes Association. Management of dyslipidemia in adults with diabetes (position statement). *Diabetes Care* 1999;22(suppl 1):S56–S59; used with permission.

Note: All lipid values are mg/dL (mmol/L).

Note: The ILIB considers a fasting TG value <150 (<1.7) desirable in both diabetic and nondiabetic patients. It concurs with the recommendations of the 1993 ADA Consensus Development Conference on the Detection and Management of Lipid Disorders in Diabetes (*Diabetes Care* 1993;16[suppl 2]:106–112) that TG-lowering intervention be initiated in primary prevention when TG is ≥200 (≥2.3), and in secondary prevention when TG is >150 (>1.7). The ILIB considers that, minimally, HDL-C <40 (<1.0) needs attention in all patients. Additionally, the ILIB recommends as a general goal in diabetic patients an LDL-C:HDL-C ratio of <3 in primary prevention and <2.5 in secondary prevention.

Table B.1-6. Priorities and Drug Choices for Treatment of Dyslipidemia in Diabetic Adults— ADA Recommendations with ILIB Comments

ADA*	ILIB Comments
I. LDL-C lowering	
First drug therapy choice: statin	Statins may be used to reduce elevated LDL-C in diabetic and nondiabetic patients. Statins also have beneficial effects on TG and HDL-C concentrations. In general, the statins have not been found to worsen glucose control in diabetes. Statins may be used to treat dyslipidemia in the presence of diabetic nephropathy with renal insufficiency. In familial forms of hypercholesterolemia, a statin may be used as monotherapy or in combination with a resin. Subset analyses of major trials have shown significant reductions in CVD events with statin therapy in diabetic patients (see text).
Second drug therapy choice: bile-acid resin or fibrate	The ILIB recommends against the use of bile-acid resins as single agents in diabetic patients. Bile-acid resins can increase VLDL TG, particularly if it is already >250 mg/dL (>2.8 mmol/L). They have little effect on HDL-C concentrations, and primarily lower TC and LDL-C concentrations. Small doses may be used as adjuvant therapy in patients with elevated VLDL TG and elevated LDL-C. In particular, resins must be used with great care if at all in the diabetic patient with GI autonomic neuropathy because they can worsen the consequences of the dysfunction (e.g., gastroparesis, constipation, fecal impaction). Resins have no adverse effects on glucose control.
II. HDL-C raising	
Drug modification is difficult except with nicotinic acid, which has a relative contraindication in diabetes, or a fibrate. Behavioral interventions such as weight loss, increased physical activity, and smoking cessation may be helpful. Maintain glycemic control.	Nicotinic acid increases insulin resistance and fasting and postprandial hyperglycemia and hyperinsulinemia. In patients with impaired glucose tolerance or an underlying tendency toward diabetes, it may accelerate the appearance of clinical diabetes. It is reserved in diabetes for refractory dyslipidemia, and used only after careful consideration and with considerable follow-up. Inability to maintain glycemic control mandates discontinuation.

Continued on next page

Table B.1-6. Priorities and Drug Choices for Treatment of Dyslipidemia in Diabetic Adults—Continued

ADA*	ILIB Comments
III. TG lowering	
First priority: glycemic control	Glycemic control may substantially reduce plasma TG.
First drug therapy choice: fibrate	Fibrates substantially lower TG and substantially increase HDL-C. The effect on LDL-C is variable but generally small. In general, the fibrates have not been found to worsen glucose control in diabetes, and some studies have suggested improved glucose tolerance. Fibrates should be used with caution if at all in the presence of diabetic nephropathy with renal insufficiency because of risk for myopathy.
A statin at a higher dosage may be moderately effective in TG reduction when high LDL-C is also present.	The effect of a statin on plasma TG concentration is proportional to the baseline TG value and is commensurate with the ability of the statin to lower LDL-C.
IV. Combined hyperlipidemia	
Improved glycemic control +	Glycemic control may substantially reduce plasma TG. LDL-C may decrease modestly.
...First drug therapy choice: statin at high dosage	See above comments about statins.
...Second drug therapy choice: statin + fibrate	As noted by the ADA, the combination of a statin and a fibrate may increase risk for myopathy. The ILIB recommends against combining a statin with a fibrate in diabetic patients with impaired renal function.
...Third drug therapy choice: resin + fibrate OR statin + nicotinic acid (nicotinic acid has a relative contraindication in diabetes; carefully monitor glycemic control)	As noted by the ADA, the combination of a statin with nicotinic acid may increase risk for myopathy. See also above comments about nicotinic acid.
	Although LDL-C effects are generally small, a fibrate may yield substantial decreases or increases in LDL-C and may be tried. Addition of a resin at a low dosage may be effective when LDL-C elevation persists.

*American Diabetes Association. Management of dyslipidemia in adults with diabetes (position statement). *Diabetes Care* 1999;22(suppl 2):S56–S59.

B.1.6 SUGGESTED READING

American Diabetes Association. Detection and management of lipid disorders in diabetes (consensus statement). *Diabetes Care* 1993;16(suppl 2):106–112.

American Diabetes Association. Nutrition recommendation and principles for people with diabetes mellitus (position statement). *Diabetes Care* 1999;22(suppl 1):S42–S45.

American Diabetes Association. Management of dyslipidemia in adults with diabetes (position statement). *Diabetes Care* 1999;22(suppl 1):S56–S59.

Assmann G, Schulte H. The Prospective Cardiovascular Münster (PROCAM) study: Prevalence of hyperlipidemia in persons with hypertension and/or diabetes mellitus and the relationship to coronary heart disease. *Am Heart J* 1988;116:1713–1724.

Austin MA, Edwards KL. Small, dense low density lipoproteins, the insulin resistance syndrome and non-insulin-dependent diabetes. *Curr Opin Lipidol* 1996;7:167–171.

The Diabetes Control and Complications Trial Research Group. The effect of intensive treatment of diabetes on the development and progression of long-term complications in insulin-dependent diabetes mellitus. *N Engl J Med* 1993;329:977–986.

Fagan TC, Sowers J. Type 2 diabetes mellitus: Greater cardiovascular risks and greater benefits of therapy. *Arch Intern Med* 1999;159:1033–1034.

Garg A. Management of dyslipidemia in IDDM patients. *Diabetes Care* 1994;17:224–234.

Goldberg RB, Mellies MJ, Sacks FM, et al. Cardiovascular events and their reduction with pravastatin in diabetic and glucose-intolerant myocardial infarction survivors with average cholesterol levels: Subgroup analyses in the Cholesterol and Recurrent Events (CARE) trial. The Care Investigators. *Circulation* 1998;98:2513–2519.

Grundy SM, Benjamin IJ, Burke GL, et al. Diabetes and cardiovascular disease: A statement for healthcare professionals from the American Heart Association. *Circulation* 1999;100:1134–1146.

Haffner SM. Management of dyslipidemia in adults with diabetes (technical review). *Diabetes Care* 1998;21:160–178.

Pyörälä K, Pedersen TR, Kjeksus J, et al. Cholesterol lowering with simvastatin improves prognosis of diabetic patients with coronary heart disease: A subgroup analysis of the Scandinavian Simvastatin Survival Study (4S). *Diabetes Care* 1997;20:614–620.

UK Prospective Diabetes Study 6. Complications in newly diagnosed type 2 diabetic patients and their association with different clinical and biochemical risk factors. *Diabetes Res* 1990;13:1–11.

UK Prospective Diabetes Study (UKPDS) Group. Intensive blood-glucose control with sulphonylureas or insulin compared with conventional treatment and risk of complications in patients with type 2 diabetes (UKPDS 33). *Lancet* 1998;352:837–853.

CHART B.1-1. EVALUATION AND TREATMENT OF LIPID DISORDERS IN ADULTS WITH DIABETES MELLITUS— ILIB RECOMMENDATIONS

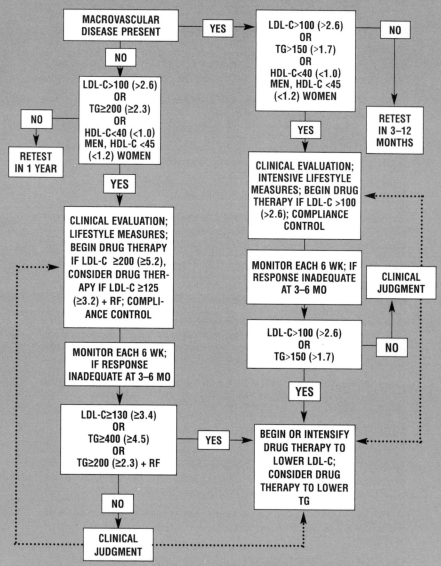

Evaluation and treatment of adults with diabetes mellitus. The ILIB algorithm combines recommendations of the 1999 ADA practice guidelines regarding LDL-C and HDL-C and recommendations of the 1993 ADA consensus panel regarding plasma TG. Annual full fasting lipoprotein analysis is recommended for patients with diabetes mellitus. HDL-C = high-density lipoprotein cholesterol; LDL-C = low-density lipoprotein cholesterol; TG = triglyceride; RF = presence of 1 or more of these risk factors: HDL-C <40 mg/dL (<1.0 mmol/L), smoking, hypertension, family history of premature CVD. All lipid values are mg/dL (mmol/L).

B.2 Management of Risk in Children and Adolescents

B.2.1 Risk Overview

The U.S. NCEP Expert Panel on Blood Cholesterol Levels in Children and Adolescents issued detailed guidelines in 1991 for the evaluation and treatment of hypercholesterolemia in young people (aged 2–19 years). The ILIB endorses the NCEP guidelines.

Dyslipidemia before adulthood is of concern because atherosclerosis begins in childhood. The **Pathobiological Determinants of Atherosclerosis in Youth** (PDAY) autopsy study of U.S. subjects aged 15–34 years correlated specific risk factors with lesion extent in particular arteries. Increased LDL-C, increased VLDL, and decreased HDL-C were associated with lesions in the aorta and right coronary artery, and smoking was associated with lesions in the abdominal aorta (McGill et al. *Arterioscler Thromb Vasc Biol* 1997;17:95–106). PDAY also found that fatty streaks and clinically significant raised lesions increase rapidly in both prevalence and extent across the age span studied (Strong et al. *JAMA* 1999;281:727–735). Children and adolescents with cholesterol elevation are more likely than their peers in the general population to have cholesterol elevation as adults. Although most youths are at only moderate risk for CHD, these will eventually account for most CHD cases among adults. True primary prevention must begin in childhood and adolescence. Identification of risk factors in a child may enable risk factor management in the entire family, because parents may change the family's lifestyle for the benefit of the child. Parents of young children often receive no routine medical care except for gynecologic care.

The population approach is the major emphasis in cholesterol control for children and adolescents and should include a low-fat, low-cholesterol diet and physical activity for all individuals in this age group.

B.2.2 Detection

In the pediatric population, screening is selective rather than universal (Table B.2-1). Lipid measurements may be performed any time after the second birthday; before then, more energy intake as fat is needed for growth, and after that age, TC and LDL-C concentrations are reasonably consistent. Screening recommendations are especially directed toward physicians who care for adults, because it is they who know the parents' risk status.

Evaluating lipids may be considered as well in a child or adolescent when a family history cannot be obtained, the patient has other risk for eventual CHD, or the patient is receiving medication that can alter lipid concentrations. As in adults, lipid determinations may be misleading if the patient is actively ill or has an infectious disease; testing should be avoided in these circumstances. Intraindividual variation in lipoprotein cholesterol values in the short term (weeks to months) is greater in children than in adults, in part because of the frequency of acute illness and because of fluctuations in eating and activity patterns.

The ILIB notes that considerable controversy still exists about whether universal opportunistic screening for hypercholesterolemia is appropriate in children and adolescents. Parental history may not be sufficient to designate younger children for selective screening because of the young age of the parents. Also to be borne in mind are lifestyle changes between generations—for example, altered diet, including shifts away from the Mediterranean diet and the westernization of traditional Asian diets; increased smoking; and decreased physical activity. There are major uncertainties in the applicability of parental history in diverse populations because of a lack of epidemiologic data. The NCEP children's panel notes that about one half of the progeny of young victims of CVD have dyslipidemia, and it cites the serious prognosis and relatively high prevalence of familial hypercholesterolemia (FH). The pathologic lesions common in childhood are of a low grade of severity and unlikely to lead to clinical sequelae for many decades, and not all hypercholesterolemic children will be hypercholesterolemic as adults. Data from the **Muscatine Study** showed that among children whose cholesterol concentrations were greater than the 90th percentile on two occasions, 25% had cholesterol <200 mg/dL (<5.2 mmol/L) at ages 20–25 years (Lauer and Clarke *JAMA* 1990;264:3034–3038).

For most children from high-risk families, the NCEP considers it sufficient to begin individualized assessment and treatment in adulthood; the cholesterol-lowering diet, recommended for the general population aged 2 years and older, and adequate physical activity are sufficient for cholesterol control in most young people. Universal cholesterol screening could lead to overuse of cholesterol-lowering drugs in childhood and adolescence, although fear of overuse of diet or drugs should not be used as a reason to exclude young people from safe and effective preventive therapies. Beyond cholesterol screening it is vital that the physician determine other CHD risk factors, including hypertension, obesity, smoking, and lack of physical exercise. Many adverse lifestyle habits begin in childhood. An integrated approach for the physician's office to cardiovascular health promotion in youth is shown in Table B.2-2.

- Emphasis on weight control in children should be on prevention because 80–90% return to their original weight percentile after weight loss efforts. About one half to three fourths of obese schoolchildren become obese adults; persistence is related to severity in childhood.

- The American Academy of Pediatrics recommends that young people limit television viewing to no more than 2 hours daily, not only because it is a sedentary activity but also because it promotes snacking. A history of the extent of television viewing and computer and video game use can provide a useful surrogate measure of physical inactivity.

- Nearly all smokers start smoking before the age of 18 years, and adverse lipid and other effects from smoking occur from passive exposure as well as from active smoking. The American Heart Association recommends that healthcare professionals 1) anticipate smoking risks associated with the child's developmental stage, 2) ask about smoking by the patient or members of the patient's family, 3) advise those who are trying, experimenting with, or smoking cigarettes to stop, 4) assist in the smoking cessation process, and 5) arrange for follow-up on smoking status.

B.2.3 Evaluation

TC and LDL-C cutpoints for pediatric patients (Table B.2-4) are lower than for adults. As in adults, cutpoints are to be interpreted flexibly, in the context of total risk. The clinical focus of the NCEP guidelines is LDL-C, and any intervention requires establishment of LDL-C elevation by at least two fasting determinations. In some families demonstrating early CHD, the inherited risk factor seems to be low HDL-C. The significance of TG elevation in children for eventual CHD risk remains uncertain.

It should be noted that initial results of **Project HeartBeat!**, a longitudinal study of the development of CVD risk factors, suggested that the fixed screening criterion of 170 mg/dL (4.4 mmol/L) for TC will identify quite variable proportions of young people at different ages as needing repeat measurements or further intervention (Labarthe et al. *Circulation* 1997;95:2636–2642). In boys, TC would be considered unacceptable in one half of those screened at age 10 years but in substantially fewer than one fourth of those screened when aged 13–18 years. The initial results of Project HeartBeat! suggest more complex patterns of change in TC concentration from ages 8 to 18 years than have been generally recognized. The 678 subjects in this U.S. study (49% female, 20% African American) were aged 8, 11, and 14 years at entry; follow-up was every 4 months for ≤4 years.

As in adults, a full clinical evaluation should be performed if the LDL-C concentration proves to be high. Possible causes of secondary dyslipidemia considered in adults are also considered in children and adolescents. Some conditions to consider in particular are overweight and use of oral contraceptives, isotretinoin, or anabolic steroids. Other conditions to consider include hypothyroidism, glycogen storage disease, cholestatic liver disease, chronic renal disease, and pregnancy. Detection of familial dyslipidemias associated with premature CHD is already crucial during childhood to retard or prevent the development and progression of atherosclerosis. The two most common familial dyslipidemias expressed as LDL-C elevation that are currently recognized in children are FH and familial combined hyperlipidemia (FCH). It has been estimated that 1 in 25 children with LDL-C higher than 130 mg/dL (3.4 mmol/L) has heterozygous FH. In FH, hypercholesterolemia is detectable at birth. Genetic dyslipidemias are discussed in detail in the report of the NCEP Expert Panel on Blood Cholesterol Levels in Children and Adolescents. Specific molecular diagnosis is currently available only for FH, but it is hoped that such diagnosis of other common lipid disorders will be possible within a few years.

B.2.4 Treatment

As discussed, the rationale for management of dyslipidemia in childhood is strong: to limit the development of atherosclerosis, to establish lifelong lifestyle habits, and to prevent the acquisition of additional risk factors. After causes of secondary dyslipidemia have been ruled out or treated, dietary therapy is the primary intervention (Table B.2-5). The diets prescribed are those used in adults; energy intake levels are selected to support growth and development and to reach or maintain desirable body weight. Consultation with a dietitian may be needed to achieve dietary compliance, which may be complicated by the early stage of psychologic development, the lack of symptoms, and the involvement of multiple caretakers. The American Heart Association (Fisher et al. *Circulation* 1997;95:2332–2333) and the American Academy of Pediatrics (*Pediatrics* 1998;101:141–147) have both endorsed the Step I Diet (prudent diet, general cholesterol-lowering diet) in children 2 years of age or older. Safety of its use has been amply demonstrated in both prospective and survey studies. Total fat intake should not be <20% in the pediatric population (American Academy of Pediatrics *Pediatrics* 1998;101:141–147). When children are placed on an intensified cholesterol-lowering diet (Step II Diet) or a weight-reducing diet, it is important to ensure adequacy of nutrients, including unsaturated fatty acids.

Pharmacotherapy may be considered in pediatric patients 10 years of age or older when LDL-C remains very high despite vigorous lifestyle intervention, especially when multiple risk factors are present. The age cutpoint reflects the fact that early lesions of atherosclerosis generally begin to occur at about age 10; however, drug therapy may be warranted in younger patients when hyperlipidemia is severe. The only lipid-regulating drugs generally recommended at present for use in children are the bile-acid sequestrants (resins). These agents have proven efficacy, relative freedom from side effects, and apparent safety when used in children and adolescents. They are usually administered with folic acid and iron supplementation in these patients. Nicotinic acid may be used in a limited number of pediatric patients, but should be administered in these patients only by a lipid specialist. The addition of nicotinic acid to a resin may be valuable when LDL-C remains very high. As an update to the NCEP pediatric guidelines, increasing data have become available on the use of statins in children and adolescents, as is discussed in more detail in ILIB case 14 (3.14). Although more clinical trial data are needed, statin therapy may be useful in pediatric patients who have failed resins and/or nicotinic acid and who have very high LDL-C values and, typically, a strong family history of premature CVD. As with nicotinic acid, use should be by lipid specialists with experience in pediatric cases. The use of drugs in pediatric patients must be individualized, and once a drug is prescribed, careful monitoring of side effects and the pediatric patient's growth and development is required.

For elevated plasma TG in pediatric patients (Table B.2-4) the ILIB recommends dietary and other lifestyle measures unless the elevation is extreme. The ILIB notes that in pediatric patients, chylomicronemia syndrome (lipoprotein lipase deficiency or apo C-II deficiency) is a cause for concern because of the danger for pancreatitis. Low HDL-C (Table B.2-4) is generally managed by lifestyle measures. In the years since the publication of the NCEP pediatric guidelines, there has been increasing recognition of the importance of the development of obesity and aspects of the cardiovascular metabolic syndrome (see 1.3.6) in young people, although the full-blown syndrome is rare in children.

B.2.5 Diabetic Patients

The American Diabetes Association (*Diabetes Care* 1998;21[suppl 21]:S23–S31) recommends that a full fasting lipoprotein profile be obtained after the diagnosis of diabetes and the establishment of glucose control in diabetic children 2 years of age or older. When lipid values are within acceptable risk levels according to NCEP guidelines for pediatric patients, they should be redetermined at least every 5 years. Abnormal or borderline values should be confirmed by repeat testing; lipid-regulating therapy as needed should follow the NCEP pediatric guidelines. The ADA recommends that blood pressure in hypertensive children with diabetes be reduced to the corresponding age-adjusted 90th percentile values.

B.2.6 SUGGESTED READING

American Academy of Pediatrics. Cholesterol in childhood. Policy statement. *Pediatrics* 1998;101:141–147.

American Academy of Pediatrics. National Cholesterol Education Program: Report of the Expert Panel on Blood Cholesterol Levels in Children and Adolescents. *Pediatrics* 1992;89:525–584.

Fisher EA, Van Horn L, McGill HC. Nutrition and children: A statement for healthcare professionals from the Nutrition Committee, American Heart Association. AHA medical/scientific statement. *Circulation* 1997;95:2332–2333.

Freedman DS, Srinivasan SR, Valdez RA, et al. Secular increases in relative weight and adiposity among children over two decades. The Bogalusa Heart Study. *Pediatrics* 1997;99:420–426.

Gidding SS, Leibel RL, Daniels S, et al. Understanding obesity in youth. A statement for healthcare professionals from the Committee on Atherosclerosis and Hypertension in the Young of the Council on Cardiovascular Disease in the Young and the Nutrition Committee, American Heart Association. AHA medical/scientific statement. *Circulation* 1996;94:3383–3387.

Gidding SS, Morgan W, Perry C, et al. Active and passive tobacco exposure: A serious pediatric health problem. A statement from the Committee on Atherosclerosis and Hypertension in Children, Council on Cardiovascular Disease in the Young, American Heart Association. AHA medical/scientific statement. *Circulation* 1994;90:2581–2590.

Humphries SE, Galton D, Nicholls P. Genetic testing for familial hypercholesterolaemia: Practical and ethical issues. *Q J Med* 1997;90:169–181.

National High Blood Pressure Education Program Working Group on Hypertension Control in Children and Adolescents. Update on the 1987 task force report on high blood pressure in children and adolescents: A working group report from the National High Blood Pressure Education Program. *Pediatrics* 1996;98:649–658.

Strong JP, Malcom GT, McMahan CA, et al. Prevalence and extent of atherosclerosis in adolescents and young adults. Implications for prevention from the Pathobiological Determinants of Atherosclerosis in Youth Study. *JAMA* 1999;281:727–735.

Strong WB, Deckelbaum RJ, Gidding SS, et al. Integrated cardiovascular health promotion in childhood: A statement for health professionals from the Subcommittee on Atherosclerosis and Hypertension in Childhood of the Council on Cardiovascular Disease in the Young, American Heart Association. *Circulation* 1992;85:1638–1650.

Strong WB, Kelder SH. Pediatric preventive cardiology. In: Manson JE, Ridker PM, Gaziano JM, et al., eds. *Prevention of Myocardial Infarction.* New York: Oxford University Press, 1996:433–459.

Tonstad S. A rational approach to treating hypercholesterolaemia in children: Weighing the risks and benefits. *Drug Safety* 1997;16:330–341.

Table B.2-1. NCEP Lipid Screening in Children and Adolescents, Aged 2–19 Years

Screening should be performed selectively.

Measure nonfasting TC (and HDL-C* if accuracy can be ensured) if parent has TC ≥240 mg/dL (≥6.2 mmol/L). Physician may choose full fasting lipoprotein analysis as the initial assessment.

Perform full fasting lipoprotein analysis if

- TC ≥200 mg/dL (≥5.2 mmol/L), or averages ≥170 mg/dL (≥4.4 mmol/L) by two measurements
  OR
- Family history of early CVD
  OR
- Parent has familial dyslipidemia*

Physician may also wish to screen if

- Family history is unobtainable
  OR
- Other risk is present (e.g., smoking, hypertension, excess fat consumption, overweight, diabetes mellitus)
  OR
- Patient is taking medication that can alter lipid concentrations (e.g., isotretinoin, corticosteroids, anabolic steroids, anticonvulsants, high-dose estrogen)

Source: Data from American Academy of Pediatrics. National Cholesterol Education Program: Report of the Expert Panel on Blood Cholesterol Levels in Children and Adolescents. *Pediatrics* 1992;89:525–584.

*ILIB addition to NCEP recommendations. The addition of HDL-C in screening is in accordance with the ATP II guidelines, which appeared after the pediatric guidelines.

Table B.2-2. Pediatric Cardiovascular Health Schedule: Recommendations of the American Heart Association Council on Cardiovascular Disease in the Young

Age	Actions
Birth	• Obtain family history; if positive for early CVD or hyperlipidemia, introduce risk factor information, parental referral • Start growth chart • Parental smoking history → smoking cessation referral
0–2 yr	• Update family history, growth chart • With introduction of solid foods, begin teaching about healthy diet (nutritionally adequate, low in saturated fat, low in sodium) • Recommend healthy snacks as finger foods • Change to whole milk from formula or breastfeeding at ~1 yr of age
2–6 yr	• Update family history, growth chart → review growth chart with family (concept of weight for height*) • Introduce prudent diet, including ≤30% of energy intake from total fat (but not <20% for the pediatric population†), 8–10% of energy intake as saturated fat • Change to low-fat milk • Start blood pressure chart at ~3 yr of age‡; review concept of lower sodium intake • Encourage parent–child play that develops coordination • Lipid determination in child if parent has hypercholesterolemia, familial dyslipidemia, or family history of premature CVD → initiate lifestyle changes if abnormal
6–10 yr	• Update family history, blood pressure, and growth charts • Complete cardiovascular health profile of child: family history, smoking history, blood pressure percentile, weight for height, lipid determination in indicated patients, level of fitness/activity • Reinforce prudent diet and begin active antismoking counseling • Introduce fitness for health → life sport activities for child and family • Discuss role of television viewing, video games, and computer use in sedentary lifestyle and obesity
>10 yr	• Update family history, blood pressure and growth charts annually • Review prudent diet, risks of smoking, fitness benefits whenever possible • Lipid profile in indicated patients • Fitness review of personal cardiovascular health status

Source: Strong WB, Kelder SH. Pediatric preventive cardiology. In: Manson JE, Ridker PM, Gaziano JM, et al., eds. *Prevention of Myocardial Infarction.* New York: Oxford University Press, 1996:433–459; used with permission.

*Obesity is defined as ≥130% ideal body weight for height, 30 kg/m² (adolescents), or the 95th percentile or greater for subscapular skinfolds.

†American Academy of Pediatrics *Pediatrics* 1998;101:141–147.

‡If 3 consecutive interval blood pressure measurements exceed 95th percentile (Table B.2-3) and blood pressure is not explained by weight for height, diagnosis of hypertension should be made and appropriate evaluation considered.

Table B.2-3. JNC VI 95th Percentile of Blood Pressure According to Selected Ages in Girls and Boys

Age (yr)	Girls' SBP/DBP in mm Hg		Boys' SBP/DBP in mm Hg	
	50th Percentile for Height	75th Percentile for Height	50th Percentile for Height	75th Percentile for Height
1	104/58	105/59	102/57	104/58
6	111/73	112/73	114/74	115/75
12	123/80	124/81	123/81	125/82
17	129/84	130/85	136/87	138/88

Source: National Institutes of Health. *The Sixth Report of the Joint National Committee on Prevention, Detection, Evaluation, and Treatment of High Blood Pressure.* NIH publication no. 98-4080. Bethesda, MD: National Institutes of Health, 1997.

Table B.2-4. NCEP Lipid Cutpoints in Children and Adolescents, Aged 2–19 Years

Lipid	Values in mg/dL (mmol/L)
TC	
High	≥200 (≥5.2)
Borderline-high	170–199 (4.4–5.1)
Acceptable	<170 (<4.4)
LDL-C	
High	≥130 (≥3.4)*
Borderline-high	110–129 (2.8–3.3)
Acceptable	<110 (<2.8)
HDL-C	
Low	<35 (<0.9)
TG	
Quite elevated[†]	>150 (>1.7)
Moderately elevated	Males: Approx. 120 (1.4)
	Females: Approx. 130 (1.5)

Source: Data from American Academy of Pediatrics. National Cholesterol Education Program: Report of the Expert Panel on Blood Cholesterol Levels in Children and Adolescents. *Pediatrics* 1992;89:525–584.

*Approximately the 90th to 95th percentile among prepubertal children.

†The EAS notes that in pediatric patients, TG >200 mg/dL (>2.3 mmol/L) is often related to obesity, and TG >500 mg/dL (>5.6 mmol/L) is usually due to a genetic disorder.

Table B.2-5. NCEP Treatment of Hypercholesterolemia in Children and Adolescents, Aged 2–19 Years

LDL-C in mg/dL (mmol/L)*	Action†
<110 (<2.8)	**Counsel** on healthy diet and on risk factor reduction; repeat lipoprotein analysis within 5 years.
110–129 (2.8–3.3)	**Provide cholesterol-lowering diet (Step I Diet)** and other risk factor intervention; reevaluate status in 1 year.
≥130 (≥3.4)	**Perform full clinical evaluation** (family history, physical examination, laboratory tests); assess for causes of secondary dyslipidemia and for familial disorders. Some patients with familial disorders will require referral to a lipid specialist. Screen family members.
	Initiate dietary therapy and other risk reduction.
	Monitor at 6 weeks and 3 months by lipoprotein analysis. If LDL-C goal not achieved at 3 months, intensify diet, with follow-up at 3 months; if LDL-C goal not achieved at this 6-month follow-up, consider drug therapy as below.
Refractory ≥190 (≥4.9) **OR** Refractory ≥160 (≥4.1) + either positive family history of early CVD or ≥2 other persistent risk factors‡	**Consider bile-acid resin to supplement diet in patients ≥10 years of age.** The ILIB notes that it is usual to provide folic acid and iron supplementation with resins in these patients, and that nicotinic acid or statins may be used in a very limited number of pediatric patients, but only by a lipid specialist.
	Monitor at 6 weeks and then every 3 months by lipoprotein analysis; every 6 months to 1 year after LDL-C goal achieved.

LDL-C GOAL OF DIET OR OF DIET + DRUG THERAPY: <130 (<3.4), ideally <110 (<2.8)

Source: Data from American Academy of Pediatrics. National Cholesterol Education Program: Report of the Expert Panel on Blood Cholesterol Levels in Children and Adolescents. Pediatrics 1992;89:525–584.

*For intervention: established by the average of at least 2 consecutive fasting determinations.

†See Table 2.8-1 for cholesterol-lowering diet; energy intake levels in children and adolescents are to promote normal growth and development and to reach or maintain desirable body weight.

‡The NCEP notes that cutpoints that minimize misclassification between pediatric patients with and without FH are about 164 mg/dL (4.2 mmol/L) for LDL-C and 235 mg/dL (6.1 mmol/L) for TC.

B.3 Special Considerations in Women

B.3.1 Risk Overview

Historically, relatively little attention has been given specifically to CHD risk reduction in women. Yet CHD is the leading cause of death among women in many developed nations, including the United States. Vigilant management of CHD risk in women is imperative. Most women perceive their risk for cancer as much greater than their risk for CHD or stroke, although, for example, age-adjusted death rates are about three times higher for CHD than breast cancer. It is important that physicians educate their patients about CHD risk in women in general and about individual risk. The ILIB urges increased emphasis on reducing CHD risk in women.

Preventive efforts are particularly important because excess early mortality after MI in women has been reported from a number of studies, even after adjustment for age and other variables. Women have delayed hospital arrival time and have been reported to receive less aggressive care, fewer procedures, and less medication for CHD. Because of sex differences in presentation and diminished accuracy of some diagnostic tools, the diagnosis of CHD presents a greater challenge in women. Compared with men, women suffering acute MI are more likely to experience (in addition to chest pain) shoulder and neck pain, nausea and vomiting, dyspnea, or fatigue. These differences may largely reflect women's older age at presentation. Women with chronic stable angina are more likely than men to have chest pain while resting, sleeping, or under mental stress. Clinical history is considered inadequate to differentiate anginal and nonanginal chest pain in women. ECG stress testing has lower sensitivity and specificity in women, and ERT may induce a false-positive ST segment depression. Radionuclide ventriculography is of limited prognostic value in women; exercise echocardiography may be valuable. Studies have shown that physicians are less likely to recommend cardiac rehabilitation to women than men despite similar severity of disease and even though women achieve as much if not more benefit from cardiac rehabilitation.

The lack of research attention to CHD risk in women stems in part from the substantially lower absolute risk for CHD among premenopausal nondiabetic women compared with men the same age; the advent of clinical disease is delayed about 6–10 years, and the advent of MI about 20 years, in nondiabetic women compared with men. Higher LDL-C targets may be used in many premenopausal women. For example, the ATP II notes that lipid-lowering pharmacotherapy may often be delayed in pre-menopausal women when LDL-C does not exceed 220 mg/dL (5.7 mmol/L) and other risk is absent.

B.3.2 Risk Factors

Changes in lipid concentrations at menopause likely account at least in part for the increased incidence of CHD after menopause. At menopause, LDL-C concentrations rise, and may thereafter slightly exceed concentrations in men; HDL-C concentrations may decrease somewhat, but they generally remain higher in women than in men throughout life. TG concentrations rise gradually in both males and females after puberty, but at a slower rate in women; in middle age, they may decrease in men yet continue to rise in women.

Although women appear to have all the same CHD risk factors as men, there is some evidence that HDL-C and TG concentrations, as well as diabetes mellitus, play a larger role in CHD risk in women. In observational epidemiologic studies, an increase of 1 mg/dL (0.03 mmol/L) in HDL-C has been associated with a 3% decrease in CHD risk in women compared with a 2% decrease in CHD risk in men. The increase in CHD risk with rising TG is much steeper in women than in men. Meta-analysis showed risk to be increased 76% in women and 32% in men with an 88.5 mg/dL (1.0 mmol/L) rise in fasting TG (Hokanson and Austin *J Cardiovasc Risk* 1996;3:213–219). An American Heart Association/American College of Cardiology consensus panel noted that in women the optimal HDL-C concentration may be higher (≥45 mg/dL, or ≥1.2 mmol/L) and the optimal fasting TG concentration may be lower (≤150 mg/dL, or ≤1.7 mmol/L) (Mosca et al. *Circulation* 1999;99:2480–2484) than is recommended by the ATP II (i.e., HDL-C >35 mg/dL and TG <200 mg/dL) for both sexes. Diabetic women do not share their nondiabetic peers' relative premenopausal protection from CHD. According to **Framingham Study** data, a high TC:HDL-C ratio may also attenuate the premenopausal CHD advantage, as may LV hypertrophy (Kannel and Wilson *Arch Intern Med* 1995;155:57–61). Half of all CHD events in women have been associated with smoking. Moderate alcohol use in women as in men is associated with reduced risk for CHD. Women appear to be more sensitive to the toxic effects of alcohol on striated muscle and are more susceptible to alcoholic liver disease. Heavy alcohol use and breast cancer risk are associated in most studies, and alcohol use and ERT appear to increase breast cancer risk synergistically. The American Heart Association and Joint National Committee (JNC VI) recommend that women limit alcohol intake to ≤1 alcoholic drink per day, and pregnant women should not drink alcohol (Mosca et al. *Circulation* 1999;99:2480–2484; National Institutes of Health *Arch Intern Med* 1997;157:2413–2446).

The clinician should be aware that oral contraceptive use can greatly increase CVD risk in women who smoke; this risk increases with age, particularly after age 35, and with heavy smoking. The American Heart Association recommends that women with a family history of premature CVD have lipid analysis before taking oral contraceptives, and that women with significant risk factors for diabetes have glucose testing before taking them (Mosca et al. *Circulation* 1999;99:2480–2484). The third-generation-progestogen, low-dose oral contraceptives have very little effect on lipid or glucose metabolism. Current oral contraceptive formulations continue to increase risk for high blood pressure; risk decreases quickly with discontinuation.

B.3.2.1 Data from Clinical Trials of Lipid-Regulating Interventions

In cholesterol-lowering trials with clinical event endpoints in which results in women have been analyzed separately, benefit in women generally equaled or even exceeded that in men. Data in secondary prevention are available from the clinical endpoint statin trials. In the **Scandinavian Simvastatin Survival Study** (4S), the 34% reduction in major coronary events with therapy was the same as that in men, and need for revascularization was reduced 49% in women, compared with 41% in men. There were too few deaths in the subset of women to allow meaningful analysis of their all-cause death rates, although the investigators considered it highly likely that significant benefit will be found in an appropriately powered trial (Miettinen et al. *Circulation* 1997;96:4211–4218). In the **Cholesterol and Recurrent Events** (CARE) trial, pravastatin therapy yielded early reduction of a wide range of CVD events in post-MI women with average cholesterol concentrations, including reductions in coronary death or nonfatal MI (43%), combined coronary events (46%), PTCA (48%), CABG (40%), and stroke (56%). Risk reductions in women tended to be greater than in men (respective reductions of 21%, 20%, 18%, 24%, and 25% in the CARE men) (Lewis et al. *J Am Coll Cardiol* 1998;32:140–146). In the **Long-term Intervention with Pravastatin in Ischemic Disease** (LIPID) trial, conducted in patients with a wide range of baseline cholesterol values, there was no significant heterogeneity between benefits of pravastatin therapy in women and men (LIPID Study Group *N Engl J Med* 1998;339:1349–1357). The **Air Force/Texas Coronary Atherosclerosis Prevention Study** (AFCAPS/TexCAPS), testing lovastatin, was the first large-scale primary-prevention trial of LDL-C lowering to include a substantial number of women. Risk for a first major coronary event was reduced 46% in these postmenopausal, generally healthy women, compared with 37% in the men, although the small numbers of events among the women precluded statistical significance (Downs et al. *JAMA* 1998;279:1615–1622). Although additional studies should be a priority, these subset analyses provide strong support for aggressive cholesterol-lowering therapy in women with and without atherosclerotic disease.

In addition, angiographically monitored secondary-prevention trials (see 1.6) that analyzed vascular results separately in women found significant coronary benefit in this subgroup, including the **Canadian Coronary Atherosclerosis Intervention Trial** (CCAIT) of lovastatin (Waters et al. *Circulation* 1995;92:2404–2410), the **University of California, San Francisco, Arteriosclerosis Specialized Center of Research (UCSF-SCOR) Intervention Trial** of combination-drug therapy in heterozygous FH (Kane et al. *JAMA* 1990;264:3007–3012), and the **Program on the Surgical Control of the Hyperlipidemias** (POSCH) using partial ileal bypass surgery (Buchwald et al. *Ann Surg* 1992;216:389–398). In the **Post Coronary Artery Bypass Graft** (Post-CABG) trial of aggressive cholesterol-lowering drug therapy, decreased risk with therapy for progression in saphenous vein grafts did not differ between women and men despite a greater number of risk factors in women (Campeau et al. *Circulation* 1999;99:3241–3247).

In a number of studies of lifestyle interventions, lipid responses were less strong in women than in men. There is no evidence that the efficacy or adverse effect profiles of lipid-regulating drugs are different in women.

B.3.3 Pregnancy

During pregnancy, plasma TG rises gradually, paralleling estrogen increases. Its values are doubled or tripled at term and return to prepregnancy concentrations at about 6 weeks postpartum. Pancreatitis during pregnancy is uncommon. Most cases are caused by cholelithiasis; few (4–6%) are linked to hyperlipidemia. LDL-C initially drops during pregnancy; after about 8 weeks, it rises to about a 50–60% increase at term, remaining elevated for up to 8 weeks after delivery. HDL_2 increases to about a twofold peak at midgestation, then falls, remaining at term about 15% above baseline. It is not clear whether repeated exposure to the lipid changes of pregnancy increases risk for atherosclerosis. A patient with latent hyperlipidemia may be identified by hyperlipidemia in pregnancy, although postpartum lipid determinations should be postponed for 6 months in women who were not dyslipidemic before pregnancy.

Because safety of use in pregnancy is not proved, lipid-regulating drugs are customarily discontinued when possible before conception. Women with significant hyperlipidemia should be advised to bear children over a limited number of years. Bile-acid resins are particularly appropriate for women considering pregnancy. In 134 women with inadvertent exposure to lovastatin or simvastatin at therapeutic dosages, no relation was found between exposure and the occurrence of adverse pregnancy outcomes (Manson et al. *Reprod Toxicol* 1996;10:439–446).

B.3.4 Postmenopausal Hormone-Replacement Therapy

Beginning at age 40 or as requested, all women should be counseled about the potential benefits and risks of hormone-replacement therapy. Many large observational epidemiologic studies have demonstrated that postmenopausal oral ERT is associated with lower risk for CHD. In 10-year data from the observational **Nurses' Health Study**, current estrogen use was associated with a 44% decrease in risk for CHD as well as a 39% decrease in risk for cardiovascular death (Stampfer et al. *N Engl J Med* 1991;325:756–762). Risk for stroke appears to be similar in users and nonusers.

The first interventional results are now available, from the **Heart and Estrogen–Progestin Replacement Study** (HERS), conducted in 2,763 postmenopausal women with CHD (Hulley et al. *JAMA* 1998;280:605–613). At 4-year follow-up, those assigned to conjugated equine estrogens plus medroxyprogesterone acetate (Prempro) versus placebo had an increased relative risk for nonfatal MI or CHD death during the first year (RR 1.52) and decreased risk during years 4 and 5 (RR 0.67). Risks for thrombo-embolic events and gallbladder disease were significantly higher with hormone use. Hormone therapy decreased LDL-C 11% and increased HDL-C 10%. It is not recommended that women with CHD start this combined hormone therapy de novo for the purpose of secondary prevention, although it may be appropriate for women already receiving replacement therapy (≥1 year) to continue it while further clinical trial results are awaited. Additional trial data are needed to clarify the CHD effects of hormone-replacement therapy. Awaited with particular anticipation is completion of the primary-prevention trial that is part of the Women's Health Initiative of the U.S. National Institutes of Health. Results are anticipated by 2005.

The beneficial effects of oral estrogens on the lipoprotein profile are a likely mechanism to account for any cardioprotection. Oral estrogens (0.625 mg/day conjugated estrogen or 2 mg/day micronized estradiol) usually increase HDL-C and decrease LDL-C, each by about 15%. In addition, however, oral estrogens may significantly increase TG, particularly when TG is already elevated. Estrogens may also lower concentrations of Lp[a]. Benefits of estrogen use may relate as well to such cardioprotective factors as lower fasting blood glucose and lower blood pressure, and there is some evidence that estrogen might exert effects to protect the vascular wall from atherosclerosis that are independent of lipid metabolism. Effects of estrogen on arterial tone have been intensively investigated. Endothelial production of nitric oxide, producing vasodilation, is attenuated by menopause and restored by ERT. The selective estrogen receptor modulator raloxifene has also been shown to have beneficial effects on plasma lipid values and coagulation parameters. Raloxifene 60 or 120 mg/day lowered LDL-C by 12% and did not increase TG but also did not increase HDL-C (Walsh et al. *JAMA* 1998;279:1445–1451). No data are available, however, concerning raloxifene and CHD risk.

The clinician may consider oral ERT for control of dyslipidemia in post-menopausal women. In some cases, ERT may obviate use of lipid-regulating agents. Transcutaneously administered estrogens appear to have less effect on lipoprotein concentrations. Exogenous estrogens do not have a U.S. Food and Drug Administration indication for lowering lipids or reducing

CHD risk. If estrogen administration increases TG markedly, the estrogen should probably be discontinued. Combining ERT and a statin may retain the HDL-C-raising effect of estrogen and the LDL-C-lowering effect of the statin while keeping TG at baseline (Davidson et al. *Arch Intern Med* 1997;157:1186–1192).

Concomitant progestin administration reduces or eliminates the increased risk for endometrial cancer with estrogen use. There is far less information about the effects of the combined use of estrogen and progestin on either CHD risk or lipoproteins, although it appears that the combination blocks some of the harmful lipid effects of progestin while allowing the beneficial lipid effects of estrogen to persist. Adherence to standard recommendations for breast cancer screening is prudent when ERT is used.

For symptoms of menopause, tibolone, a synthetic steroid with estrogenic, androgenic, and progestogenic properties, appears to be at least as efficacious as other forms of hormone-replacement therapy. Used in women with at least 1 year of amenorrhea, tibolone does not cause withdrawal bleeding. The agent's androgenic action may be responsible for the reported decreases in fasting TG and Lp[a] but also for the decreases in HDL-C. Most available data indicate that tibolone has no significant effect on LDL-C concentration. Whether use of tibolone will be associated with decreased cardiovascular risk is unknown, but it has been speculated that demonstrated positive effects on vascular reactivity and to some extent on fibrinolysis may counterbalance potentially deleterious effects on the lipid profile. No data are available on prevention of fractures with tibolone, although effects on markers of bone metabolism and bone mass appear to be similar to those of other forms of hormone-replacement therapy.

The decision to treat with hormone-replacement therapy must take into account menopausal symptoms and risks for CHD, osteoporosis, cancer, deep vein thrombosis, and pulmonary embolism (Table B.3-1). The balance between risks and benefits needs to be carefully assessed. As noted above, it does not appear to be advisable on the basis of HERS results to start combination therapy de novo in women with established CHD.

B.3.5 SUGGESTED READING

Buchwald H, Campos CT, Matts JP, et al. Women in the POSCH trial: Effects of aggressive cholesterol modification in women with coronary heart disease. *Ann Surg* 1992;216:389–398.

Douglas PS, Ginsburg GS. The evaluation of chest pain in women. *N Engl J Med* 1996;334:1311–1315.

Hulley S, Grady D, Bush T, et al. Randomized trial of estrogen plus progestin for secondary prevention of coronary heart disease in postmenopausal women. Heart and Estrogen/progestin Replacement Study (HERS) Research Group. *JAMA* 1998;280:605–613.

LaRosa JC. Cholesterol management in women and the elderly. *J Intern Med* 1997;241:307–316.

Lewis SJ, Sacks FM, Mitchell JS, et al. Effect of pravastatin on cardiovascular events in women after myocardial infarction: The Cholesterol and Recurrent Events (CARE) trial. *J Am Coll Cardiol* 1998;32:140–146.

Limacher MC. Exercise and rehabilitation in women: Indications and outcomes. *Cardiol Clin* 1998;16:27–36.

Limacher MC. The role of hormone replacement therapy in preventing coronary artery disease in women. *Curr Opin Cardiol* 1998;13:139–144.

Miettinen TA, Pyörälä K, Olsson AG, et al., for the Scandinavian Simvastatin Study Group. Cholesterol-lowering therapy in women and elderly patients with myocardial infarction or angina pectoris: Findings from the Scandinavian Simvastatin Survival Study (4S). *Circulation* 1997;96:4211–4218.

Mosca L, Grundy SM, Judelson D, et al. Guide to preventive cardiology for women. AHA/ACC scientific statement: Consensus panel statement. *Circulation* 1999;99:2480–2484.

Mosca L, Manson JE, Sutherland SE, et al. Cardiovascular disease in women: A statement for healthcare professionals from the American Heart Association. AHA medical/scientific statement. *Circulation* 1997;96:2468–2482.

Rich-Edwards JW, Manson JE, Hennekens CH, et al. The primary prevention of coronary heart disease in women. *N Engl J Med* 1995;332:1758–1766.

Roger VL, Gersh BJ. Myocardial infarction. In: Julian DG, Wenger NK, eds. *Women and Heart Disease*. St. Louis: Mosby, 1997:135–150.

Waters D, Higginson L, Gladstone P, et al. Effects of cholesterol lowering on the progression of coronary atherosclerosis in women. A Canadian Coronary Atherosclerosis Intervention Trial (CCAIT) substudy. *Circulation* 1995;92:2404–2410.

Table B.3-1. Possible Benefits and Risks of Hormone-Replacement Therapy

	Hormone Therapy Regimen	
	Estrogen Alone	**Estrogen plus Progestin**
Possible Benefits		
CHD	May decrease risk by 35%	May decrease risk by 20–35%, but less information than for estrogen alone
		May increase risk during first year in women with CHD
Fractures due to osteoporosis	May decrease risk for hip fracture by 25%	Same, but less information than for estrogen alone
Menopausal symptoms	Fewer hot flashes and other symptoms of menopause	Same
Bladder function	Fewer bladder problems	Same
Cognitive function	Some evidence for prevention of onset of dementia and improvement of symptoms in the established condition	
Possible Risks		
Breast cancer	May increase risk for breast cancer by 25%	Same, but less information than for estrogen alone
Uterine cancer	May increase risk	No known increase in risk
Blood clots	May increase risk in legs or lungs	Same
Side effects and vaginal bleeding	More period-like symptoms	Same

Source: Modified from Grady D, Rubin SM, Petitti DB, et al. Hormone therapy to prevent disease and prolong life in postmenopausal women. *Ann Intern Med* 1992;117:1016–1037; used with permission.

B.4 Special Considerations in the Elderly

B.4.1 Risk Overview

The absolute risk for morbidity and mortality from CVD rises steeply with age. In the United States, people who are 65 or older, two thirds of whom are women, account for nearly 60% of hospital admissions for acute MI, and 85% of CHD deaths are in this age group. In men peak prevalence of CHD has shifted to the elderly years with the success of CHD risk interventions in the middle-aged, and in women CHD is largely a postmenopausal disease.

B.4.2 Risk Factors

The major risk factors for CHD continue to operate beyond age 60 and even beyond age 70 in both men and women. Cigarette smoking remains a powerful risk factor throughout life, whether in terms of relative or attributable risk, perhaps because it, apparently, predisposes to plaque rupture. There is no evidence that the pathobiology of atherothrombosis differs among age groups. Neither does the risk from hypertension decline with age; in fact, the elderly are more susceptible to its deleterious effects. Isolated systolic hypertension may develop at older ages, and, particularly among older individuals, SBP is a better predictor of CVD events than is DBP. The **Systolic Hypertension in the Elderly Program** showed reduced incidence of both stroke and MI in the elderly receiving antihypertensive therapy (SHEP Cooperative Research Group *JAMA* 1991;265:3255–3264). LV hypertrophy is an important CHD risk factor often overlooked in the elderly. CHD produced by diabetes mellitus appears to increase as aging progresses.

The continued risk includes the risk of dyslipidemia. Relative risk for CHD has been shown to be increased by hypercholesterolemia in many although not all studies in the elderly, and the risk relation has included those >80 years of age. There may be some diminution in relative risk from elevated cholesterol as the elderly age, although not all analyses support weakened predictivity. Nevertheless, the absolute risk attributable to hypercholesterolemia increases with age because of the much higher absolute risk for a CHD event in older people. Plasma TG and, in particular, HDL-C also predict CHD risk in the elderly. In a large prospective cohort study of elderly men and women, HDL-C <35 mg/dL (<0.9 mmol/L) compared with HDL-C ≥60 mg/dL (≥1.6) quadrupled the relative risk for CHD death among people aged 71–80 and doubled that risk among people older than 80 (Corti et al. *JAMA* 1995;274:539–544).

B.4.2.1 Data from Clinical Trials of Lipid-Regulating Drugs

Findings from lipid-regulating clinical trials limited to subjects >65 years of age are not available. However, subset analyses of trial data strongly support the efficacy and safety of cholesterol-lowering therapy in the young elderly (ages 60–75), and it would seem reasonable to extrapolate the results to even older individuals. By 2000, individual patient data on more than 60,000 subjects, including 20,000 elderly subjects, should be available from the **Cholesterol Treatment Trialists' Collaboration** (Cholesterol Treatment Trialists' Collaboration *Am J Cardiol* 1995;75:1130–1134).

In secondary prevention, subset analysis in the **Stockholm Ischemic Heart Disease Secondary Prevention Study** showed similar CHD benefit from combined clofibrate and nicotinic acid therapy in younger subjects and subjects 60–69 years of age at the trial's beginning (Carlson and Rosenhamer *Acta Med Scand* 1988;223:405–418). More recent data are available from clinical endpoint trials of statins and of gemfibrozil (Table B.4-1); see 1.5 for trial overviews. In the **Scandinavian Simvastatin Survival Study** (4S), statin therapy significantly reduced all-cause mortality (34%), CHD mortality (43%), major coronary events (34%), and need for revascularization (41%) in 518 hypercholesterolemic men and women who were ≥65 years of age at enrollment (70–76 years of age at the end of the study) (Miettinen et al. *Circulation* 1997;96:4211–4218). Although fewer older patients required dosage titration from 20 to 40 mg/day, lipid effects and relative risk reductions were similar in younger and older patients, consistent with other findings suggesting enhanced response to statin therapy with increasing age. In the placebo group of 4S, all-cause and CHD mortality rates in patients ≥65 years were more than twice those in patients <65 years; thus, the absolute risk reduction in these rates with therapy was more than doubled in older patients. A similar approximate doubling in reduction of absolute risk in older men and women occurred with pravastatin therapy at lower cholesterol concentrations in the **Cholesterol and Recurrent Events** (CARE) trial (Sacks et al. *N Engl J Med* 1996;335:1001–1009). Among the 640 older patients (aged 65–75 years at entry) in the CARE drug group, there were significant risk reductions in major coronary events (-32%), CHD death (-45%), and stroke (-40%). Only 11 older patients needed to be treated for 5 years to prevent a major coronary event, and only 22 to prevent a coronary death (Lewis et al. *Ann Intern Med* 1998;129:681–689). In the **Long-term Intervention with Pravastatin in Ischemic Disease** (LIPID) trial, across a wide range of entry cholesterol values, clinical benefit extended to the 1,081 men and women in the pravastatin group who at enrollment were 65–69 years of age (CHD risk reduced 28%) and to the 660 who at enrollment were 70–75 years of age (CHD risk reduced 15%) (LIPID Study Group *N Engl J Med* 1998;339:1349–1357). There was no evidence of significant heterogeneity of treatment effect in any prespecified subgroup in LIPID.

CVD benefit was achieved in elderly men with multiple coexisting illnesses in the **Veterans Affairs Cooperative Studies Program High-Density Lipoprotein Cholesterol Intervention Trial** (HIT) through gemfibrozil therapy that raised HDL-C and lowered plasma TG without lowering LDL-C (Rubins et al. *N Engl J Med* 1999;341:410–418). Angiographic trials have shown that even advanced disease responds to cholesterol lowering, so it is not too late to begin therapy in the elderly. In the **Post Coronary Artery Bypass Graft** (Post-CABG) trial, aggressive cholesterol-lowering drug therapy delayed the progression of atherosclerosis in saphenous vein grafts in men and women 60–74 years of age at enrollment as well as in younger patients (Campeau et al. *Circulation* 1999;99:3241–3247).

In primary prevention, subset analyses of data from the **West of Scotland Coronary Prevention Study** (WOSCOPS) and the **Air Force/Texas Coronary Atherosclerosis Prevention Study** (AFCAPS/TexCAPS) support extension of benefit to older patients. In both of these statin trials, as in 4S, CARE, and LIPID, statin therapy was well tolerated by older patients and there were low rates of adverse effects. WOSCOPS enrolled hypercholesterolemic men aged 45–64 years, 3,370 of whom were 55 years of age or older. In this older group, pravastatin therapy reduced the rate of nonfatal MI and CHD death by a significant 27%, compared with a significant 40% in the younger men (Shepherd et al. *N Engl J Med* 1995;333:1301–1307). Subsequent analysis showed higher coronary event rates in the older group (West of Scotland Coronary Prevention Group *Lancet* 1996;348:1339–1342). In the primary-prevention WOSCOPS hypercholesterolemic men aged 55–64 years who had at least one additional risk factor, 5-year absolute risk for a coronary event exceeded 10% (2%/year). This level of risk would make them candidates for aggressive risk factor reduction, including lipid-lowering drug therapy, according to Second Joint (European) Task Force recommendations (*Eur Heart J* 1998;19:1434–1503); see Figure A.2-1. Lovastatin therapy in AFCAPS/TexCAPS, conducted in generally healthy older men and women with average cholesterol and below-average HDL-C concentrations, appeared to attenuate the risk conferred by age and sex, among other risk factors (Downs et al. *JAMA* 1998;279:1615–1622). Age was analyzed in AFCAPS/TexCAPS according to whether it was above or below the baseline median (57 in men and 62 in women; upper limit 73).

B.4.3 Diagnosis and Evaluation

Hypothyroidism is a common cause of secondary dyslipidemia in the elderly. It should be considered in elderly hypercholesterolemic patients even when other symptoms and signs are lacking; classic clinical features are often absent in the hypothyroid in this age group. Thyroid hormone replacement should be used cautiously in patients with CHD to avoid precipitating acute MI or precipitating or aggravating ventricular arrhythmias, angina, or congestive heart failure. In both sexes in the elderly, moderately elevated TC may be due to increased HDL-C, in which case no treatment is needed.

CHD is often undiagnosed or misdiagnosed in the elderly. Classic angina pectoris is a less common feature in this age group, and atypical angina is common. Many elderly people may not experience exertional angina because of a sedentary lifestyle. Angina may be misdiagnosed as peptic ulcer disease or degenerative joint disease. Symptoms of acute MI may be atypical or very vague; acute MI should be suspected when there are unexplained behavior changes, acute signs of cerebral insufficiency, or dyspnea. As many as 60% of MIs in the very elderly may be unrecognized or clinically silent.

THE ILIB LIPID HANDBOOK: APPENDIXES

B.4.4 Treatment

It is inappropriate to exclude the elderly from cholesterol lowering simply on the basis of age. High-risk but otherwise healthy elderly patients are candidates for lipid-lowering therapy. Intervention is justified for individuals with reasonable life expectancy, and good quality of life is a relative indication. Beginning lipid-lowering therapy as primary prevention in those >75 years is an issue of debate, but therapy begun in earlier years should be continued. Beginning intervention in the older elderly requires appropriate judgment. Practical considerations include motivation and understanding, food preferences and nutritional soundness, cost of drugs, potential for drug interactions, choice of antihypertensive therapy, and renal function monitoring. Target lipid concentrations in the elderly are those used for the general adult population.

Smoking cessation, treatment of hypertension, weight reduction in the obese, and increased physical activity should also be pursued. Because the elderly often have multiple medical problems, several factors must be balanced in making treatment decisions. In a longitudinal study conducted in the middle-aged and elderly, the preselected stratification variables of BMI, exercise pattern, and smoking predicted subsequent disability (Vita et al. *N Engl J Med* 1998;338:1035–1041). Better health habits postponed disability more than 5 years and compressed it into fewer years at the end of life.

Certain causes of secondary hypertension such as primary aldosteronism may occur more frequently among the elderly. Blood pressure must be measured with care in this age group because some have pseudohypertension due to vascular stiffness. Starting dosages of antihypertensive agents should be about half those used in younger patients. Blood pressure goals are the same as in younger patients (<140/90 mm Hg), although an interim goal of SBP <160 mm Hg may be necessary in patients with marked systolic hypertension. Other recommendations for control of hypertension in the elderly can be found in the report by the U.S. National High Blood Pressure Education Program Working Group on Hypertension in the Elderly (*Hypertension* 1994;23:275–285).

There is no evidence that slight overweight in the elderly requires correction. It is never too late to begin exercising; an important noncoronary benefit is increase in bone density. Current exercise recommendations— which emphasize the importance of total amount of exercise, cite the

benefits of intermittent exercise, and advocate lower-intensity exercise—
are particularly relevant to the elderly. Brisk walking constitutes a substantial percentage of the lower maximal oxygen uptake in the elderly.
Older patients should be cautioned to reduce the intensity of their exercise
in hot or humid conditions because of reduced efficiency of temperature
regulation, and more time should be allotted for warm-up and cool-down
activities. Clinical features have been defined to identify patients who
should have ECG monitoring during exercise.

B.4.4.1 Cholesterol-Lowering Dietary Therapy

According to surveys, the elderly are concerned about and willing to make
lifestyle changes to maintain health. Changes in diet appear to be as effective in the elderly as in the middle-aged for improving the lipid profile.
Dietary therapy needs to be carefully individualized (e.g., to accommodate
rigid food preferences), particularly because elderly patients may be at risk
for malnutrition because of isolation, depression, poverty, or coexisting
diseases. An intensified cholesterol-lowering diet (Step II Diet) may not be
advisable for all elderly patients, and some elderly people may overcomply
with diet, leading to caloric deficiency, calcium deficiency, or constipation
or even bowel obstruction from excessive intake of fiber.

B.4.4.2 Lipid-Regulating Drug Therapy

Particular caution should be used in proceeding to lipid-regulating pharmacotherapy in the elderly. These patients are especially vulnerable to the
adverse effects of drugs. Secondary prevention is of great importance
because most patients with established atherosclerotic disease are 65 or
older, and clinical judgment is crucial in deciding whether to use aggressive therapy. The common phenomena in older patients of decreasing
body size, decreasing cardiac output, reduced renal and hepatic function,
and multiple drug therapy mandate special concern for drug interactions
and appropriate dosage. Well-tolerated lipid-lowering drugs for older
patients are the HMG-CoA reductase inhibitors (statins) and the fibric-acid
derivatives (fibrates) (Table B.4-2). Compliance approaches that may be
particularly important in older patients are moral support, simplification
of therapy, and minimization of side effects.

B.4.5 SUGGESTED READING

Aronow WS, Ahn C. Risk factors for new coronary events in a large cohort of very elderly patients with and without coronary artery disease. *Am J Cardiol* 1996;77:864–866.

Barzel US. Hypothyroidism: Diagnosis and management. *Clin Geriatr Med* 1995;11:239–249.

Corti M-C, Guralnik JM, Salive ME, et al. HDL cholesterol predicts coronary heart disease mortality in older persons. *JAMA* 1995;274:539–544.

Forman R, Aronow WS. Management of postmyocardial infarction in the elderly patient. *Clin Geriatr Med* 1996;12:169–180.

Fraser GE, Shavlik DJ. Risk factors for all-cause and coronary heart disease mortality in the oldest-old: The Adventist Health Study. *Arch Intern Med* 1997;157:2249–2258.

Grundy SM. Cholesterol lowering in the elderly population. *Arch Intern Med* 1999;159:1670–1678.

Grundy SM. The role of cholesterol management in coronary disease risk reduction in elderly patients. *Endocrinol Metab Clin North Am* 1998;27:655–675.

LaRosa JC. Dyslipidemia and coronary artery disease in the elderly. *Clin Geriatr Med* 1996;12:33–40.

LaRosa JC. Triglycerides and coronary risk in women and the elderly. *Arch Intern Med* 1997;157:961–968.

Lewis SJ, Moye LA, Sacks FM, et al. Effect of pravastatin on cardiovascular events in older patients with myocardial infarction and cholesterol levels in the average range. Results of the Cholesterol and Recurrent Events (CARE) trial. *Ann Intern Med* 1998;129:681–689.

Miettinen TA, Pyörälä K, Olsson AG, et al., for the Scandinavian Simvastatin Study Group. Cholesterol-lowering therapy in women and elderly patients with myocardial infarction or angina pectoris. Findings from the Scandinavian Simvastatin Survival Study (4S). *Circulation* 1997;96:4211–4218.

National High Blood Pressure Education Program Working Group. National High Blood Pressure Education Program Working Group report on hypertension in the elderly. *Hypertension* 1994;23:275–285.

Schaefer EJ, Lichtenstein AH, Lamon-Fava S, et al. Efficacy of a National Cholesterol Education Program Step 2 Diet in normolipidemic and hypercholesterolemic middle-aged and elderly men and women. *Arterioscler Thromb Vasc Biol* 1995;15:1079–1085.

Vita AJ, Terry RB, Hubert HB, et al. Aging, health risks, and cumulative disability. *N Engl J Med* 1998;338:1035–1041.

Wenger NK. Physical inactivity and coronary heart disease in elderly patients. *Clin Geriatr Med* 1996;12:79–88.

West of Scotland Coronary Prevention Group. West of Scotland Coronary Prevention Study: Identification of high-risk groups and comparison with other cardiovascular intervention trials. *Lancet* 1996;348:1339–1342.

Table B.4-1. Findings in Older Subjects in Recent Clinical Endpoint Trials of Lipid-Regulating Drug Therapy

Trial (Agent)	Age in Subset at Entry	N (%)	Sex	% Relative Risk Reduction with Drug Therapy	
				CHD	CHD Death
Secondary prevention					
4S (simvastatin)	65–70	1,021 (23)	M/F	34	43
CARE (pravastatin)	65–75	1,283 (31)	M/F	32	45
LIPID (pravastatin)	65–69	2,168 (24)	M/F	28	—
	70–75	1,346 (15)	M/F	15	—
HIT (gemfibrozil)	66–73	1,266 (50)	M	26*	—
Primary prevention					
WOSCOPS (pravastatin)	55–64	3,370 (51)	M	27	—
AFCAPS/TexCAPS (lovastatin)	Age above median (>57M, >62F; upper limit 73)	3,180 (48)	M/F	30	—

Note: See text for full names of trials.

*Relative risk reduction in combined secondary endpoint of CHD death, nonfatal MI, and confirmed stroke.

Table B.4-2. Notes on Treatment of Dyslipidemia in the Elderly

Therapy	Considerations
Lifestyle modification	Carefully individualize diet to ensure adequacy of nutrition. Regular physical activity if appropriate.
Drug therapy	Use particular caution in proceeding to drug therapy, because the elderly may be particularly susceptible to adverse effects. Statins and fibrates are well tolerated.
Statins	Most cases of severe myopathy have occurred in older patients, particularly those with coexisting disease, e.g., renal insufficiency.
Resins	Associated constipation may be a particular problem. Absorption of other drugs may be decreased.
Fibrates	Occurrence of gallstones may be increased; cholecystectomy carries more risk in older patients. Other possible side effects are GI distress, impotence, and, in patients with renal insufficiency, myopathy.
Niacin	Common side effects may be more pronounced, e.g., flushing, dry skin, dry mouth. Impaired glucose tolerance may be aggravated. Niacin raises uric acid concentrations and may precipitate gout.

C. CHARACTERIZING DYSLIPIDEMIA

C.1 Determining Blood Lipid Values

Table C.1-1. Selected Considerations in Blood Sampling

Consideration	Notes
Nonfasting vs. fasting	TC and HDL-C: Nonfasting acceptable in follow-up.
	TG: Fasting always required (12- to 14-hour fast; water and calorie-free liquids permitted, including tea or coffee without whitener).
Fingertip vs. venous	Screening (TC, HDL-C, TG): Fingertip blood and dry chemistry techniques may be used.
	Decision making: Follow-up testing with venous blood required.
Serum vs. plasma	Standardize sample type from one test date to the next: Plasma lipid values are about 4% lower than serum values.
	Serum: Preferably, collect blood in tubes without anticoagulant.
	Plasma: Tubes containing EDTA may be used.
Establishing baseline values	Establish baseline values by using several blood samples over 1–3 months, for estimate of variability, and use for evaluation of treatment.
	Cholesterol values normally fluctuate day to day by perhaps 3% or more. Note that seasonal variations also occur, e.g., cholesterol values modestly increase in spring and modestly decrease in autumn.
	Fluctuations from day to day of >30% occur in fasting TG independent of meal pattern.
Concurrent illness or other condition	MI: Determine lipid values within 24 hours of the onset of chest pain. Beginning about 12 hours after an MI, LDL-C values decrease for up to 12 weeks. However, decreases in lipid values generally do not exceed 10% during the first 24 hours; decreases >10% generally do not occur until ≥48 hours after admission. All patients admitted with an MI or suspected MI are fasting at some point during the first 24 hours, and fasting lipid values should be determined during that window of opportunity. After this period, deferral of diagnostic lipid evaluation for 4–6 weeks is customary.
	Other major illness or surgery: Defer for 3 months. Minor illness: Defer for 3 weeks.
	Pregnancy: Associated with physiologic hyperlipidemia; defer testing until after delivery, but test patients with history of HTG (pregnancy could elevate TG to pancreatitis range). During pregnancy, LDL-C, HDL-C, and TG rise (see also B.3.3).
Diet	Patient followed current diet for 3 weeks and maintained constant weight.

Continued on next page

Table C.1-1—*Continued*

Consideration	Notes
Posture	Standardize patient posture because posture can alter cholesterol values by changing plasma volume; patient seated for 5–10 minutes convenient. If patient lies down for 10 or 15 minutes before blood sampling, the lipid values may be lower than they otherwise would be. TG and TC are 9–19% higher when the patient is erect rather than recumbent.
Phlebotomy technique	Draw venous sample without prolonged stasis; use tourniquet as briefly as possible before inserting needle and release before drawing sample.
Laboratory	Use same laboratory for consistency over time. Seek a laboratory that participates in a reliable standardization program—in the United States, preferably one that has its lipid assays standardized through one of the National Network Laboratories of the Centers for Disease Control and Prevention. Rapid capillary blood (fingerstick) methodology for TC, TG, and HDL-C can produce satisfactory results provided determinations are standardized in the same fashion as venous serum or plasma determinations.
Recognition of chylomicronemia	Refrigerate fasting serum or plasma for 12 hours. Finding of creamy supernatant indicates presence of chylomicrons. Rule of thumb: TG >300 mg/dL (>3.4 mmol/L) confers turbidity to plasma.
Non-HDL-C	Some investigators have suggested that non-HDL-C—i.e., LDL-C + IDL-C + VLDL-C, a measure of all lipoproteins that contain apo B—is a better representation of "atherogenic cholesterol" than is LDL-C. In fasted plasma (which is usually absent chylomicrons), apo B concentrations may serve as a marker of the number of atherogenic particles, and it has been recognized as a clinical CHD predictor. The clinician may wish to be familiar with these research issues.
Limitations	At present, routine laboratory measurements cannot identify small, dense LDL, nor can they distinguish whether HTG is caused by small or large particles. IDL, VLDL, and small, dense LDL may be associated with increased risk for atherosclerosis. (Rule of thumb: A preponderance of small, dense LDL in the LDL fraction is likely when fasting TG exceeds 190 mg/dL [2.1 mmol/L]; normal LDL size is likely when fasting TG is below 105 mg/dL [1.2 mmol/L].)

Table C.1-2. Estimating LDL-C with the Friedewald Formula

Units*	Formula
Conventional (mg/dL)	LDL-C = TC − HDL-C − (TG/5)
Système International (SI) (mmol/L)	LDL-C = TC − HDL-C − (TG/2.2)

Note: **The formula does not apply if** the patient has:
- TG >400 mg/dL (>4.5 mmol/L),
- Apo E2/2 phenotype or genotype, or
- Fredrickson type III hyperlipidemia (see Tables 2.2-2 and 2.6-1).

In each of these circumstances, direct determination of LDL-C in a specialized laboratory is required for accuracy. Also, high Lp[a] diminishes the accuracy of the Friedewald formula. Ideally, the calculated LDL-C value should be adjusted to reflect the contribution of Lp[a] cholesterol: LDL-C ≈ LDL-C $_{calculated}$ − (Lp[a]/3) (in mg/dL). With enzymatic TG determination, the Friedewald formula can be used until TG values of about 700 mg/dL (8 mmol/L), except in type III hyperlipidemia.

*Conversion values: 0.02586 for cholesterol (TC, HDL-C, LDL-C) and 0.01129 for TG (as multiplier from mg/dL to mmol/L; as divisor from mmol/L to mg/dL).

C.2 Common Causes and Presentations of Hyperlipidemia

Table C.2-1. General Clinical Tips

Hyperlipidemia	Diagnostic Tips
Primary or secondary?	• Primary disorders most commonly identified in clinical practice are FCH, polygenic hypercholesterolemia, FH, and type III hyperlipidemia (see 2.6).
	• In addition to lifestyle factors (e.g., diet rich in saturated fats, excessive alcohol consumption, obesity), common causes of secondary dyslipidemia include type 2 diabetes mellitus, hypothyroidism, chronic renal failure, and nephrotic syndrome (see 2.5).
	• If dyslipidemia persists despite treatment of causes of secondary dyslipidemia, treat as primary lipid disorder.
Hypercholesterolemia	• Usually polygenic, multifactorial causes; commonly associated with excessive intake of dietary fat
	• Searching for genetic origin through specialized laboratory methods may be useful in family counseling.
Hypertriglyceridemia	• Moderate HTG common; often accompanies diabetes mellitus, central obesity, or excessive use of alcohol
	• Severe HTG usually combination of genetic factors and secondary dyslipidemia
	• HDL-C often low
	• When HTG marked, TC usually elevated, although to a smaller degree than the TG elevation
	• Isolated moderate HTG may be associated with increased risk for CHD.
	• Clinician should be aware of described, perhaps relatively common syndrome of moderate HTG and low HDL-C, often with hypertension, insulin resistance, hyperinsulinemia, higher glucose values, higher uric acid values, and microalbuminuria (overweight and moderate TC elevation may be present); increased risk for CHD with this cluster of risk factors referred to as the *cardiovascular metabolic syndrome* or *insulin resistance syndrome* (see 1.3.6)

Combined hyperlipidemia (HC + HTG)

- Establishment of specific cause usually difficult
- May be secondary to diabetes mellitus or renal disease
- Usually moderate; if TC >300 mg/dL (>7.8 mmol/L) + TG >400 mg/dL (>4.5 mmol/L), test for type III hyperlipidemia or refer to specialized center.
- Combined hyperlipidemia + low HDL-C = high risk

Look for manifestations of atherosclerosis

- For example, vascular bruits, decreased peripheral pulses

Look for manifestations of dyslipidemia

- For example, corneal arcus, xanthelasmas/xanthomas, hepatosplenomegaly

Note: See Table 2.2-2 for approximate percentages of hyperlipidemic patients (U.S.) presenting with each Fredrickson phenotype.

C.3 Obtaining Family History

Table C.3-1. Step-by-Step Family History

1.	Draw a pedigree	Index patient, parents, siblings, children, grandparents, aunts, uncles
2.	Check	Are all blood relatives?
3.	Ask	Is relative alive or dead?
	If relative is alive	How old? Any CVD? If so, at what age? Smoke? Other CVD risk factors?
	If relative has died	Age at death? Cause of death? Other major illness? If CVD present, at what age? CVD risk factors?
4.	Discard	All uncertain information
5.	Assume	Family history is uninformative but not negative for CVD if patient knows little about relatives' cardiovascular health
6.	Consider in general	Number and sex of relatives at risk Current age and age when CVD developed Additional risk factors in those positive for disease Number of expected cases of CVD given family risk factors Number of observed vs. number of expected cases
7.	Favorable family history when	Longevity in most members

Note: In general, women give a better family history than do men.

D. ELEMENTS OF LIPID-REGULATING THERAPY

D.1 Lipid Effects of Lifestyle Changes

Table D.1-1. Major Effects of Lifestyle Changes on Plasma Lipid Concentrations

Intervention	Major Lipid Benefit*		
	↓ LDL-C	↓ TG[†]	↑ HDL-C[‡]
↓ Saturated fat	√	√	
↓ Dietary cholesterol	√		
↓ Weight in overweight patients	√	√	√
↑ Physical activity	√	√	√
Stop smoking[§]			√

*Coordinate benefits of interventions include ↓ blood pressure, ↑ glucose tolerance, ↓ coronary thrombosis, possibly inherent CVD protection from weight control, exercise, consumption of fruits, vegetables, and grains. Regular moderate exercise is an important component of weight-loss programs.

[†]For HTG, ↓ alcohol beneficial in most patients; ↑ fatty fish consumption may be helpful; also emphasize smoking cessation.

[‡]Physical inactivity, obesity, and smoking are major causes of secondary decreased HDL-C.

[§]Another major beneficial effect of smoking cessation is lowering of plasma fibrinogen concentration, although this change may take many years. Some studies have reported slight decreases in LDL-C with smoking cessation. It is also important to avoid second-hand smoke.

D.2 Implementing a Heart-Healthy Diet

D.2.1 Food Choices

The cholesterol-lowering, or heart-healthy, diet (see Table 2.8-1) comprises:

- An abundance of plant foods, such as whole-grain bread and whole-grain cereals, vegetables (raw and cooked), fruit, and legumes

- Unhydrogenated vegetable oils as the principal source of fat, especially oils, such as olive oil and canola oil, rich in monounsaturated fatty acids (oleic acid)

- Nonfat and low-fat dairy products

- Fish and poultry (with skin removed)

- Lean meat and eggs (limit to no more than 4 yolks per week; egg whites may be eaten ad libitum)

The first step in helping patients make dietary changes is to assess their current eating pattern in detail. An example of a simple dietary assessment tool that can be used in a physician's office is the MEDFICTS Dietary Assessment Questionnaire, available in the full report of the ATP II (National Cholesterol Education Program *Circulation* 1994;89:1329–1445) or at www.nhlbi.nih.gov (search *medficts*). The expertise of a dietitian will be required for more accurate assessment. Next, the patient must be shown how to achieve his or her target level of saturated fat in the cholesterol-lowering diet. The recommended maximum number of grams of saturated fat varies according to energy intake (Table D.2-1). Typically, decreasing saturated fat will decrease dietary cholesterol as well; the Mediterranean diet (Table D.2-2) is an example of a diet that is usually low in saturated fat. Calories can be adjusted for weight loss or maintenance, and exercise can enhance weight loss and the effects of the cholesterol-lowering diet. A well-balanced diet that includes foods from all food groups should be emphasized.

D.2.2 Additional Dietary Issues

D.2.2.1 Dietary Treatment of HTG

Patients with HTG may need more detailed dietary guidance. Carbohydrates, saturated fat, and alcohol are all potential contributors to elevated plasma TG. In these patients, increased emphasis should be placed on raising the ratio of monounsaturated to saturated fatty acids and on increasing energy intake from complex carbohydrates without increasing energy intake from all carbohydrates. Weight reduction in the overweight is needed, physical activity should be increased, and, if possible, alcohol should be avoided completely. It may also be helpful to increase consumption of fish rich in omega-3 fatty acids. In the emergency treatment of severe HTG (TG >1,000 mg/dL, or >11.3 mmol/L), a fat-free diet should be administered for at least 3 days. In severe chylomicronemia, use medium-chain TG (available as margarine or MCT oil) and avoid long-chain TG.

D.2.2.2 Lifestyle Changes to Raise HDL-C

HDL-C is generally little affected by changes in the type of dietary fatty acids. Substitution of carbohydrates for fat can lower HDL-C concentration. The key lifestyle changes to increase HDL-C are weight loss in the overweight, increased physical activity, and smoking cessation. With smoking cessation, HDL-C increases on average 6–8 mg/dL (0.2 mmol/L); significant improvements occur quickly, within as little as 30 days.

D.2.2.3 Mediterranean Diet

The Mediterranean diet (Table D.2-2) is low in saturated fatty acids, has a high content of monounsaturated fatty acids, and is rich in complex carbohydrates and fiber. Use of the Mediterranean diet will help lower risk for CHD in primary and secondary prevention—as seen in both observational studies such as the **Seven Countries Study** (Keys et al. *Am J Epidemiol* 1986;124:903–915) and clinical trials such as the **Lyon Diet Heart Study** (de Lorgeril et al. *Circulation* 1999;99:779–785)—as well as possibly lower risk for cancer, diabetes, obesity, and hypertension. It is difficult to single out individual components beyond the low saturated fat content for the

CHD benefit, and in Mediterranean populations with low CHD risk, other factors such as a high level of physical activity and infrequent obesity likely play important roles. Examples of components of interest are olive oil, fruits and vegetables, and moderate alcohol intake.

D.2.2.4 Alcohol

Moderate alcohol consumption has a well-demonstrated cardioprotective effect. About half of the effect may be attributed to increases in HDL-C. Total mortality rate is lowest in people who consume 1 or 2 drinks per day; it rises rapidly with increasing number of drinks as they exceed 3 daily. Excessive alcohol intake is an important risk factor for hypertension, can cause resistance to antihypertensive therapy, and is a risk factor for stroke. Because of the intrinsic risks of alcohol use, it is inadvisable to issue general population guidelines recommending alcohol use.

D.2.2.5 Fish

Fish is a good source of protein and is low in saturated fat; cold-water fish are rich in omega-3 fatty acids, which lower plasma TG and may improve the coagulation profile, promote the vasodilation mediated by endothelium-derived nitric oxide, and have an antiarrhythmic effect, among other favorable effects. General use of fish oil supplementation (which should be considered drug therapy) is not recommended.

D.2.2.6 Soluble Fiber

As part of a low-fat diet, foods rich in soluble fiber (e.g., barley, oats, beans, soy products, guar gum, and pectin found in apples, cranberries, currants, and gooseberries) can help maximize lowering of plasma cholesterol.

D.2.2.7 Soy Protein

Many studies have demonstrated that substituting soy protein for animal protein lowers cholesterol concentrations. Soy contains an appreciable amount of isoflavones; a growing body of evidence suggests that phytoestrogens may confer health benefits related to CVD, cancer, osteoporosis, and menopausal symptoms.

D.2.2.8 Vitamins Affecting Homocysteine Concentration

Evidence is insufficient to recommend homocysteine measurements in the general population, but physicians may wish to consider measurements in patients with premature CHD or stroke who do not have classic risk factors and in patients with a history of venous thromboembolism and atherosclerosis. When the homocysteine concentration exceeds 12 µmol/L, the patient should be encouraged to increase intake of foods rich in folic acid, including oatmeal, (low-fat or nonfat) milk and milk products, green leafy vegetables, oranges, and bananas. Daily supplements of 400–800 µg folic acid + 2–4 mg vitamin B6 + 400 µg vitamin B12 may be given. Supplements in these dosages should always be considered when the homocysteine concentration exceeds 30 µmol/L.

D.2.2.9 Antioxidant Vitamin Supplementation

Results from clinical trials testing dietary antioxidant supplementation are mixed. It is recommended that antioxidant vitamins and other nutrients be derived from foods, not supplements. Good sources of antioxidant vitamins include fresh vegetables, whole-grain cereal, native olive oil, canola (rapeseed) oil, fruit, and green tea.

D.2.2.10 Plant Stanols/Sterols

As part of the diet, plant (or phyto-) stanols—and to a lesser degree their parent compounds, plant sterols—lower plasma cholesterol concentrations because of their ability to reduce absorption of cholesterol in the intestine. Plant stanol ester foods (e.g., margarine-like spreads) were introduced into markets in the 1990s and are clinically proven, effective tools for the dietary management of hypercholesterolemia. Consumption of 2–3 g daily of plant stanols in foods containing plant stanol esters may be expected to decrease LDL-C by about 15%. LDL-C lowering is the chief lipid effect; there are not significant effects on TG and HDL-C concentrations. With an action entirely in the GI tract, stanol esters are well tolerated and apparently free of side effects. Thus, the use of plant stanols can augment cholesterol management with currently recommended diets.

D.2.3 SUGGESTED READING

Appel LJ, Moore TJ, Obarzanek E, et al., for The Dash Collaborative Research Group. A clinical trial of the effects of dietary patterns on blood pressure. *N Engl J Med* 1997;336:1117–1124.

Ascherio A, Willett WC. Health effects of trans fatty acids. *Am J Clin Nutr* 1997;66(4 suppl):1006S–1010S.

Assmann G, de Backer G, Bagnara S, et al. International consensus statement on olive oil and the Mediterranean diet: Implications for health in Europe. *Eur J Cancer Prev* 1997;6:418–421.

Denke MA. Cholesterol-lowering diets: A review of the evidence. *Arch Intern Med* 1995;155:17–26.

Food and Agriculture Organization. *Fats and Oils in Human Nutrition: Report of a Joint Expert Consultation (WHO.FAO).* FAO Paper 57. Geneva: World Health Organization, 1994.

Krauss RM, Deckelbaum RJ, Ernst N, et al. Dietary guidelines for healthy American adults: A statement for health professionals from the Nutrition Committee, American Heart Association. *Circulation* 1996;94:1795–1800.

Kris-Etherton PM, for the Nutrition Committee. Monounsaturated fatty acids and risk of cardiovascular disease. AHA science advisory. *Circulation* 1999;100:1253–1258.

Kushi LH, Lenart EB, Willett WC. Health implications of Mediterranean diets in light of contemporary knowledge. 2. Meat, wine, fats, and oils. *Am J Clin Nutr* 1995;61(suppl):1416S–1427S.

Lichtenstein AH, Van Horn L. Very low fat diets. *Circulation* 1998;98:935–939.

Pearson TA. Alcohol and heart disease. AHA science advisory. *Am J Clin Nutr* 1997;65:1567–1569.

Schaefer EJ, Lamon-Fava, Ausman LM, et al. Individual variability in lipoprotein cholesterol response to National Cholesterol Education Program Step 2 diets. *Am J Clin Nutr* 1997;65:823–830.

Stone NJ. Fish consumption, fish oil, lipids, and coronary heart disease. *Circulation* 1996;94:2337–2340.

Stone NJ, Nicolosi RJ, Kris-Etherton P, et al. AHA conference proceedings. Summary of the Scientific Conference on the Efficacy of Hypocholesterolemic Dietary Interventions. American Heart Association. *Circulation* 1996;94:3388–3391.

Tribble DL. Antioxidant consumption and risk of coronary heart disease: Emphasis on vitamin C, vitamin E, and beta-carotene. A statement for healthcare professionals from the American Heart Association. *Circulation* 1999;99:591–595.

Van Horn L. Fiber, lipids, and coronary heart disease. A statement for healthcare professionals from the Nutrition Committee, American Heart Association. *Circulation* 1997;95:2701–2704.

Table D.2-1. Grams of Fat and Saturated Fat According to Energy Intake

Calorie Level	Grams of Fat Equal to 30% of Calories	Grams of Saturated Fat Equal to 10% of Calories	Grams of Saturated Fat Equal to 7% of Calories
1,200	40	13	9
1,400	47	16	11
1,600	53	18	12
1,800	60	20	14
2,000	67	22	16
2,200	73	24	17
2,400	80	27	19
2,600	87	29	20
2,800	93	31	22
3,000	100	33	23

Note: Nutrition calorie = kilocalorie; 1 kcal = 4.184 kJ.

Note: To approximate calories needed per day to maintain an ideal weight, multiply the ideal weight in pounds avoirdupois by 11 calories if the individual is nearly sedentary, 13 calories if the individual is moderately active, 15 calories if the individual is a moderate exerciser or a physical worker, or 18 calories if the individual is an extremely active exerciser (1 lb avdp = 0.454 kg).

Table D.2-2. Key Components of the Mediterranean Diet

- High intake and variety of fruits, vegetables, legumes, and grains
  - —Fresh fruit with meals as dessert

- High ratio of monounsaturated to saturated fatty acids
  - —Olive oil as principal source of fat

- Moderate consumption of milk and dairy products
  - —Principally as cheese and yogurt*

- Enhanced consumption of fish and poultry†

- Low intake of red meat and meat products‡

- 0–4 egg yolks consumed weekly

- Alcohol consumption at moderate levels
  - —Typically with meals and mainly in the form of wine

*Choose skim milk, low-fat cheese, and fat-free yogurt.
†Prepare without skin.
‡Choose lean meat.

D.3 Management of Overweight and Obesity

Table D.3-1. World Health Organization Classification of Overweight and Obesity in Adults

Category	BMI (kg/m²)*	Risk for Comorbidities†
Underweight	<18.5	Low (but risk for other clinical problems increased)
Normal weight	18.5–24.9	Average
Overweight	≥25.0	
Pre-obese	25.0–29.9	Increased
Obese class I	30.0–34.9	Moderate
Obese class II	35.0–39.9	Severe
Obese class III	≥40.0	Very severe

Source: World Health Organization. *Obesity: Preventing and Managing the Global Epidemic. Report of a WHO Consultation on Obesity, June 1997.* Geneva: World Health Organization, 1998.

Note: The BMI values are age and sex independent. BMI, however, may not correspond to the same degree of fatness between populations, in part because of different body proportions.

ILIB note: Although BMI has great clinical utility, raised BMI, which can result from a large mass of muscle or bone, does not automatically indicate a high degree of adiposity.

ILIB note: The same overweight and obesity class cutpoints are used in the U.S. National Institutes of Health guidelines (*Clinical Guidelines on the Identification, Evaluation, and Treatment of Overweight and Obesity in Adults.* Bethesda, MD: National Institutes of Health, 1998).

*Nonmetric conversion formula = [weight (lb)/height (in)²] x 704.5.

†Risk can be affected by a range of factors, for example, nature of the diet, ethnic group, and activity level. A measure of fat distribution (e.g., waist circumference, waist:hip ratio) is also important in calculating risk (see Table D.3-2). Risks associated with increasing BMI begin at BMI <25.0 and are continuous and graded. Risks may differ among populations.

Table D.3-2. Modification of the Risk of Obesity by Waist Circumference in Caucasians (World Health Organization)

Risk for Obesity-Associated Metabolic Complications	Waist Circumference in cm (in)	
	M	F
Increased	≥94 (37)	≥80 (32)
Substantially increased	≥102 (40)	≥88 (35)

Source: Modified in format from World Health Organization. *Obesity: Preventing and Managing the Global Epidemic. Report of a WHO Consultation on Obesity, June 1997.* Geneva: World Health Organization, 1998.

Note: The identification of risk by using waist circumference will be population specific, and risk depends as well on degree of obesity and other risk factors, including type 2 diabetes mellitus. The issue is under investigation.

ILIB note: The U.S. National Institutes of Health guidelines (1998) also endorse increased risk according to the waist circumference of ≥102 cm in men and ≥88 cm in women.

Table D.3-3. BMI for Selected Heights and Weights

Body Weight in kg (lb)

Height in cm (in)	BMI 25	BMI 27	BMI 30
147 (58)	54 (119)	59 (129)	65 (143)
150 (59)	56 (124)	60 (133)	67 (148)
152 (60)	58 (128)	63 (138)	69 (153)
155 (61)	60 (132)	65 (143)	72 (158)
158 (62)	62 (136)	67 (147)	74 (164)
160 (63)	64 (141)	69 (152)	77 (169)
163 (64)	66 (145)	71 (157)	79 (174)
165 (65)	68 (150)	73 (162)	82 (180)
168 (66)	70 (155)	76 (167)	84 (186)
170 (67)	72 (159)	78 (172)	87 (191)
173 (68)	74 (164)	80 (177)	89 (197)
175 (69)	77 (169)	83 (182)	92 (203)
178 (70)	79 (174)	85 (188)	94 (207)
180 (71)	81 (179)	87 (193)	98 (215)
183 (72)	83 (184)	90 (199)	100 (221)
185 (73)	86 (189)	93 (204)	103 (227)
188 (74)	88 (194)	95 (210)	106 (233)
191 (75)	91 (200)	98 (216)	109 (240)
193 (76)	93 (205)	100 (221)	112 (246)

Source: National Institutes of Health. *Clinical Guidelines on the Identification, Evaluation, and Treatment of Overweight and Obesity in Adults.* Bethesda, MD: National Institutes of Health, 1998.

Table D.3-4. U.S. National Institutes of Health Recommendations for Weight Loss in Adults

Most successful strategies:

Calorie reduction—Reducing dietary fat without reducing calorie intake will not lead to weight loss; however, reducing dietary fat is a practical way to reduce calories. In dietary fat reduction, priority should be given to reduction of saturated fatty acids (low SFA intake is needed even in individuals of normal weight to help prevent atherosclerosis). It is often helpful for the patient to begin a meal with a helping of very low calorie or bulky food, such as clear soup or a mixed or green salad with very little or no oil.

Increased physical activity—Patients should engage in moderate physical activity, progressing to ≥30 minutes on most or preferably all days of the week (see D.4). Exercise enables preferential loss of fat with preservation of lean tissue and may suppress the appetite. Significant weight loss should not be expected with exercise alone without calorie restriction.

Behavior therapy—Designed to improve eating and physical activity habits. Specific behavior therapy strategies include self-monitoring, stress management, stimulus control, problem solving, contingency management, cognitive restructuring, and social support. Many self-help and commercial diet programs are available. However, commercial programs often use "crash diets," which are almost always unsuccessful. To enhance compliance, the physician plays a supportive, encouraging role, seeing the patient as often as is practicable. A registered dietitian or other health professional can play an important role.

Initial goal: Reduce body weight by ~10% from baseline, an amount that reduces obesity-related risk factors. With success, further weight loss, if warranted, may be attempted.

Time line: Six months of therapy for a 10% reduction in body weight, with a weight loss of 0.5–1 kg (1–2 lb) per week (calorie deficit of 500–1,000 kcal/day). Patience and persistence are needed, but the outcome may be very rewarding.

Weight maintenance: A priority after the first 6 months of weight loss therapy. Rate of weight loss usually declines and weight plateaus after 6 months because of reduced energy expenditure at the lower weight.

Drug therapy: Lifestyle therapy should be tried for at least 6 months before consideration of physician-prescribed drug therapy. Weight loss drugs approved for long-term use may be tried as part of a comprehensive weight loss program that includes dietary therapy and physical activity in carefully selected patients (BMI >30 kg/m^2 without additional risk factors; BMI >27 kg/m^2 with ≥2 other risk factors) who have been unable to lose weight or maintain weight loss with conventional nondrug therapies. Disorders considered important enough to warrant drug therapy at a BMI of 27–29.9 are hypertension, dyslipidemia, CHD, type 2 diabetes, and sleep apnea. Drug therapy may also be used during the weight maintenance phase of treatment. Drug safety and effectiveness beyond 1 year of total treatment have not been established.

Surgery: Weight loss surgery is an option for carefully selected patients with clinically severe obesity (BMI >40 kg/m^2, or BMI >35 kg/m^2 with comorbid conditions) when less invasive methods have failed and the patient is at high risk for obesity-associated illness. Lifelong medical surveillance after surgery is required.

Nonparticipants: Overweight or obese patients who do not wish to lose weight, or who are not candidates for weight loss treatment, should be counseled on strategies to avoid further weight gain.

Older patients: Age alone should not preclude weight loss treatment in older adults. Management should be guided by careful evaluation of risks and benefits.

Source: Adapted from National Institutes of Health. *Clinical Guidelines on the Identification, Evaluation, and Treatment of Overweight and Obesity in Adults.* Bethesda, MD: National Institutes of Health, 1998.

ILIB note: Prevention of weight gain with aging among adults is a high priority, especially given the difficulty of weight loss. Fundamental modifications in eating and exercise habits must be made as young adults progress toward middle age.

D.4 Exercise Recommendations

Table D.4-1. American Heart Association Exercise Recommendations: Key Points

NEED

Primary and secondary prevention of CVD. Individuals of all ages should be physically active.

ASSESSMENT

Assess every patient's customary physical activity level as an integral part of the medical history.

PRESCRIPTION

With the support of other health professionals, prescribe and give advice about physical activity with individual patient needs and capabilities in mind. Emphasize the risks of a sedentary lifestyle.

TYPE AND AMOUNT OF ACTIVITY*

In selecting the level of exercise, the foremost consideration is the individual's overall health status. Medical evaluation, including exercise testing, is needed for some individuals, although not for the apparently healthy individual <40 years of age who has no coronary risk factors and who plans to begin only a moderate-intensity activity program.

Most benefit against risk for CVD death can be achieved through moderate-intensity activity. It is recommended that the activity be performed for at least 30–60 minutes 4–6 times per week or 30 minutes on most days of the week. Activities are best preceded by warm-up and followed by cool-down. Frequency, duration, and intensity should be individualized according to personal satisfaction, mode, and progression. Patients who meet the daily standards may gain additional health and fitness benefit by becoming more active or including more vigorous activity.

Exercise should include aerobic activities such as bicycling (stationary or routine), swimming, and other active recreational/leisure sports. Brisk, regular walking is a readily accessible form of exercise for achieving aerobic fitness. The exercise program should additionally include resistive exercises, performed 2–3 times weekly using free weights or standard equipment.

Some health benefit can be achieved even by low-intensity activities performed daily.

FOLLOW-UP

Follow-up needs to be systematic. Maintenance of the exercise program may be the greatest challenge. Identify barriers.

POTENTIAL RISKS

Potential risks of physical activity can be reduced by medical evaluation, risk stratification, supervision, and education. Among individuals who require physician consultation before beginning or increasing physical activity are those with a known or suspected cardiovascular, respiratory, metabolic, orthopedic, or neurologic disorder. Exercise testing can be an important basis for appropriate prescription of physical activity.

Continued on next page

**ILIB note:* A factor to consider in the prescription is the prior activity level of the patient. It is unrealistic, for example, to instruct a completely sedentary patient to exercise for 30 minutes 3 times a week at 60–70% of maximal capacity; a more gradual approach would be advisable.

Table D.4-1—*Continued*

CARDIAC REHABILITATION

Recommend medically supervised exercise programs in some cases. Avoid bias against women, which has been described.

ADDITIONAL CONSIDERATIONS IN SECONDARY PREVENTION

Exercise Testing
Required before a physical activity program is begun.

Symptom-limited exercise testing is often performed as soon as the patient's condition has stabilized (as early as 2–6 weeks after the coronary event). If echocardiography, angiography, or other studies are not indicated, a regular conditioning program can be initiated with a careful prescription of activity based on results of the exercise test.

Type of Activity
In the first 2 weeks after MI or CABG, emphasis is offsetting the effects of bed rest or former periods of inactivity. Activity should increase when the patient's condition is stable, as determined by ECG, vital signs, and symptomatic standards. Precautions include awareness of chest discomfort, faintness, and dyspnea. Initial activities need to be supervised.

Unless the individual can attend supervised classes where other activities can be provided, walking is recommended for early activity. Walking should at first be limited, then gradually increase to 5–10 minutes of continuous movement. Active but nonresistive range-of-motion of upper extremities is also well tolerated as long as healing of a sternal incision is not stressed or impaired.

For purposes of conditioning, large-muscle group activities should be performed for at least 20–30 minutes at least 3–4 times weekly. Activities should be preceded by warm-up and followed by cool-down. Supervised group sessions are recommended initially. Unsupervised home programs are acceptable in motivated, low-risk individuals who understand the basic principles of exercise training.

Sources: Data from:

Fletcher GF, Balady G, Blair SN, et al. Statement on exercise. Benefits and recommendations for physical activity programs for all Americans. A statement for health professionals by the Committee on Exercise and Cardiac Rehabilitation of the Council on Clinical Cardiology, American Heart Association. *Circulation* 1996;94:857–862.

Fletcher GF. How to implement physical activity in primary and secondary prevention. A statement for healthcare-professionals from the Task Force on Risk Reduction, American Heart Association. *Circulation* 1997;96:355–357.

Table D.4-2. EAS Exercise Recommendations

Description of Exercise	Amount
1. Set target heart rate	Heart rates suitable for normal individuals:
	Age 20–29 115–145
	Age 30–39 110–140
	Age 40–49 105–130
	Age 50–59 100–125
	Age 60–69 95–120
	Not for those taking cardiac drugs; may need to be modified in light of ECG findings. Heart rates represent 60–75% of maximum rates.
2. Warm up	5–10 minutes stretching and range-of-motion exercises
3. Aerobic phase: Walking or hiking, jogging, treadmill, stationary bicycle, bicycling, swimming, rowing, cross-country skiing, aerobic dancing, stair climbing, calisthenics, or calisthenics with lifting of light weights	
If done 4–5 times/week	20–30 minutes
If done 2–3 times/week	45–60 minutes
4. Cool down	5–10 minutes gradual decrease in exercise intensity

Continued on next page

Table D.4-2—Continued

Supervision of Exercise*	Supervision Requirements
1. Low-risk individuals	Optional
2. Individuals >35 years of age, with CHD or at high risk for CHD	Exercise ECG to determine suitable exercise level
3. High-risk individuals (e.g., impaired LV function, high-grade arrhythmia, exercise-induced ischemia or hypotension, persistently excessive heart rate during exercise)[†]	Medically supervised exercise, often with ECG monitoring, at least initially[†]

Source: Data from International Task Force. Prevention of coronary heart disease: Scientific background and new clinical guidelines. Recommendations of the International Task Force for Prevention of Coronary Heart Disease. *Nutr Metab Cardiovasc Dis* 1992;2:113–156.

*It is important that individuals learn to perform exercises properly, both to minimize risk for injury and to maximize results. Brisk walking is especially suitable in the unsupervised category, and is suitable for previously sedentary coronary patients and for the elderly. The physician should ask the patient to report any coughing, faint-ness, or chest pain that occurs during exercise. Guidelines for exercise testing have been published by the European Society of Cardiology Working Group on Exercise Physiology, Physiopathology and Electrocardiography (*Eur Heart J* 1993;14:969–988). Detailed recommendations on exercise rehabilitation in cardiac patients have been formulated by the Working Group on Cardiac Rehabilitation of the European Society of Cardiology (*Eur Heart J* 1992;13(suppl C):1–45) as well as by Horgan et al. (*Br Heart J* 1992;67:412–418). Guidelines from the Preventive and Rehabilitative Exercise Committee of the American College of Sports Medicine appear in: Mahler DA. *Guidelines for Exercise Testing and Prescription*, ed. 5. Malvern, PA: Williams and Wilkins, 1994. American Heart Association guidelines appear in: Fletcher GF, Balady G, Froelicher VF, et al. Exercise standards: A statement for healthcare professionals from the American Heart Association. *Circulation* 1995;91:580–615, and Pina IL, Balady GJ, Hanson P, et al. Guidelines for clinical exercise testing laboratories. A statement for healthcare professionals from the Committee on Exercise and Cardiac Rehabilitation, American Heart Association. *Circulation* 1995;91:912–921.

[†]More detailed classifications, by the American Heart Association, are given in Table D.4-3.

Table D.4-3. American Heart Association Physical Activity Classifications

Class A

Definition

Apparently healthy individuals. No evidence of increased CVD risk with exercise

Individuals included

1) <40 years with no symptoms or known presence of CHD or major CHD risk factors; 2) any age with no symptoms or known presence of CHD or major CHD risk factors and with normal exercise test

Activity guidelines

No restrictions other than basic guidelines:
1) Exercise only when feeling well. 2) Do not exercise vigorously soon after eating. 3) Adjust exercise to the weather. 4) Slow down for hills. 5) Wear proper clothing and shoes. 6) Understand personal limitations. 7) Select appropriate exercises. 8) Be alert for symptoms such as discomfort in the upper body, faintness, shortness of breath, and discomfort in bones and joints. 9) Watch for signs of overexercising: inability to finish, inability to converse during the activity, faintness or nausea after exercise, chronic fatigue, sleeplessness, or aches and pains in the joints. 10) Start slowly and progress gradually.

ECG and blood pressure monitoring

Not required

Supervision required

None

Class B

Definition

Known, stable CVD with low risk from vigorous exercise but slightly greater risk than in class A. Moderate activity not believed to be associated with increased risk

Individuals included

1) CHD (MI, CABG, PTCA, angina pectoris, abnormal exercise test, abnormal coronary angiograms), stable condition, clinical characteristics outlined next; 2) valvular heart disease; 3) congenital heart disease; 4) cardiomyopathy; 5) exercise test abnormalities that do not meet criteria outlined in class C

Clinical characteristics

1) New York Heart Association class I or II; 2) exercise capacity >6 METs; 3) no evidence of heart failure; 4) free of ischemia or angina at rest or on the exercise test ≤6 METs; 5) appropriate rise in SBP during exercise; 6) no sequential ectopic ventricular contractions; 7) satisfactory ability to self-monitor intensity of activity

Activity guidelines

Activity individualized with exercise prescription by qualified personnel trained in basic cardiopulmonary resuscitation or with electronic monitoring at home

ECG and blood pressure monitoring

Only during the early prescription phase of training, usually 6–12 sessions

Supervision required

Medical supervision during prescription sessions and nonmedical supervision for other exercise sessions until the individual understands how to monitor activity

Continued on next page

Table D.4-3—Continued

Class C

Definition

Moderate to high risk for cardiac complications of exercise and/or unable to self-regulate activity or to understand recommended activity level

Individuals included

1) CHD with clinical characteristics outlined next; 2) cardiomyopathy; 3) valvular heart disease: 4) exercise test abnormalities not directly related to ischemia; 5) previous episode of ventricular fibrillation or cardiac arrest that did not occur in the presence of an acute ischemic event or cardiac procedure; 6) complex ventricular arrhythmias that are uncontrolled at mild or moderate work intensities with medication; 7) 3-vessel disease or left main disease; 8) low ejection fraction (<30%)

Clinical characteristics

1) ≥2 MIs; 2) New York Heart Association class III or greater; 3) exercise capacity <6 METs; 4) ischemic horizontal or downsloping ST depression ≥4 mm or angina during exercise; 5) fall in SBP with exercise; 6) a medical problem that the physician believes may be life threatening; 7) previous episode of primary cardiac arrest; 8) ventricular tachycardia at workload <6 METs

Activity guidelines

Activity should be individualized with exercise prescription by qualified personnel

ECG and blood pressure monitoring

Continuous during exercise until safety is established, usually in 6–12 sessions or more

Supervision required

Medical supervision during all exercise sessions until safety is established

Class D

Definition

Unstable disease with activity restriction

Individuals included

1) Unstable ischemia; 2) heart failure that is not compensated; 3) uncontrolled arrhythmias; 4) severe and symptomatic aortic stenosis; 5) other conditions that could be aggravated by exercise

Activity guidelines

No activity is recommended for conditioning purposes. Attention should be directed to treating the patient and restoring him or her to status of class C or higher. Daily activities must be prescribed on the basis of individual assessment by the patient's personal physician

Source: Data from Fletcher GF, Balady G, Froelicher VF, et al. Exercise standards: A statement for healthcare professionals from the American Heart Association. *Circulation* 1995;91:580–615.

Note: MET = metabolic equivalent (3.5 mL/kg/minute oxygen uptake).

Note: Classifications do not consider accompanying morbidities, such as type 1 diabetes, morbid obesity, severe pulmonary disease, or debilitating neurologic or orthopedic conditions, that may necessitate closer supervision during training sessions.

Note: For minimum conditioning, leisure-time activity should consume a minimum of 700 kilocalories (2,900 kJ)/week; the activity should be performed on 3 or more nonconsecutive days. Incremental benefits appear to accrue up to 2,000 kilocalories (8,400 kJ)/week (20 miles of walking or jogging). Walking appears to be as beneficial as more vigorous activities. It appears that some benefit is obtained from as little as 20 minutes of low-intensity exercise performed 3 times per week,

D.5 Smoking Cessation

Table D.5-1. Smoking Cessation: A Guide for Primary-Care Physicians

In addition to assisting patients to stop smoking, advise all patients to avoid second-hand smoke and encourage nonsmokers not to start smoking.

Brief Individual Counseling *(1–3 minutes)*

- To succeed in quitting, the smoker must want to stop, and must be able to deal with the dependence on nicotine and on the smoking habit.

- Ask about and record every patient's smoking habits, including the amount smoked and duration of the habit. A specific smoke card is of value. A hospitalized patient or a patient seen in the office for CVD or a respiratory disease provides a captive audience.

- At every subsequent visit, ask about and record current smoking habits.

- Ask about the desire to quit smoking. Concentrate efforts on patients who wish to quit.

- To enhance motivation, spell out the hazards of continued smoking and emphasize the health advantages of quitting. Be specific and encouraging; discount previous failures. Provide appropriate literature, although person-to-person contact appears to be a key determinant of effectiveness.

- Give explicit advice to quit. Brief advice is better than no advice. Even simple words of advice can be effective. The words chosen are no less a therapeutic agent than a pharmacologic agent prescribed. Training may improve the effectiveness of healthcare providers.

Extended Counseling

- For persistent smokers, trained personnel can provide more extensive counseling, or the patient may be enrolled in a special program.

- The more intense the treatment, the more effective it is. Ideally, 4–7 person-to-person sessions (≥20–30 minutes each) over 8 weeks.

- Counseling sessions yield higher cessation rates if they include general problem solving/skills training (e.g., how to resist cues to smoke) and provider support.

Modifying the Environment

- Quitters should identify and, when possible, avoid situations that trigger smoking (e.g., sitting in the smoking section of a restaurant, socializing with smokers, drinking alcohol). Alcohol avoidance during the first few weeks can be critical.

Continued on next page

Table D.5-1—*Continued*

Nicotine Replacement Therapy

- NRT can be of value in the motivated patient, but must be accompanied by the counseling program.

- Simply prescribing therapy does not constitute NRT and is usually ineffective. Essential elements are diagnosis, rational dosing, appropriate instruction, and follow-up.

- Higher than standard doses of gum or patches have not been shown to increase abstinence rates in the long-term, nor has a combination of gum and patch.

- Despite anecdotal reports of worsened unstable angina, fatal and nonfatal MIs, and stroke with use of nicotine patches, reviews and trials of transdermal nicotine suggest that NRT does not increase the already increased CVD risk of smokers. Trials included smokers with CHD or other CVD. Nevertheless, caution with NRT should be used if patients have had severe or worsening angina, a recent MI, recent cerebrovascular accident, arrhythmia, very high blood pressure, or diabetes mellitus requiring insulin. Physicians should consult product information for complete lists of contraindications and cautions.

Bupropion

- Sustained-release bupropion HCl tablets were approved by the U.S. Food and Drug Administration in May 1996 as the first non-nicotine prescription medication available for use as an aid in smoking cessation. Use is to accompany nonpharmacologic interventions. Physicians should review full product information for complete prescribing information.

- Long-term quit rates appear equivalent to those achieved with NRT (approximate doubling of smoking cessation rates at 6–12 months compared with placebo).

Acupuncture and Hypnosis

- Patients may ask about nonstandard approaches. In methodologically sound studies of acupuncture in this application, cessation rates have been low and similar to placebo. Effectiveness is also unproved for group or individual hypnosis for smoking cessation.

Source: Modified from International Task Force for Prevention of Coronary Heart Disease. *Guidelines of the European Atherosclerosis Society: A Desktop Guide to the Management of Risk Factors for Coronary Heart Disease.* London: Current Medical Literature Ltd., 1993; used with permission. Some of the additional information is from Agency for Health Care Policy and Research. *Smoking Cessation.* Clinical Practice Guidelines no. 18. AHCPR publication no. 96-0692. *Smoking Cessation: A Guide for Primary Care Clinicians.* AHCPR publication no. 96-0693. Rockville, MD: U.S. Department of Health and Human Services, 1996. Available: www.ahcpr.gov.

D.6 Lipid-Regulating Pharmacotherapy

D.6.1 Available Agents

The available classes of lipid-regulating drugs are:

- HMG-CoA reductase inhibitors (statins)
- Bile-acid sequestrants (resins)
- Fibric-acid derivatives (fibrates)
- Nicotinic acid (niacin)

These options allow drug therapy to be tailored to the specific lipid abnormality of an individual patient. Each class offers a favorable risk:benefit ratio and has well-defined effects on the major lipid fractions, although individual responses can vary. It is of great interest that the drugs' benefits possibly extend beyond their effects on lipid concentrations alone.

Oral estrogen-replacement therapy may also be considered in postmenopausal women to lower LDL-C moderately and/or to increase HDL-C moderately.

When fish oil is used as a dietary supplement to lower TG, it should be considered a drug. In general, fish-oil supplementation is not recommended, although it may have a role in the management of severe refractory HTG (in particular in the chylomicronemia of type V hyperlipidemia or after antiprotease therapy).

See 2.2.2 for definitions of Fredrickson phenotypes, Table 2.6-1 for primary dyslipidemias, and 2.9 for consideration and selection of drug therapy.

Read in conjunction with manufacturers' product information sheets. In some countries, the dosage recommendations may vary; consult product labeling.

Table D.6-1. HMG-CoA Reductase Inhibitors (Statins)

Highly effective in all conditions in which LDL-C elevation is the predominant phenotype; suitable first-line agents in FH; may be useful in type III hyperlipidemia when resistant to fibrates or niacin; well tolerated

- Statins enhance catabolism of LDL. Inhibition of hepatic HMG-CoA reductase decreases hepatic cholesterol concentration, thereby activating SREBPs (see E.1.1) and increasing the expression of LDL receptors. It has been speculated that the effect of decreased plasma TG (VLDL) may be through increased uptake of VLDL and IDL by the up-regulated LDL (apo B/E) receptors and that blocked cholesterol biosynthesis makes less cholesterol available for VLDL production. The mechanism for increased HDL-C is unknown

- Moderate effects in lowering TG. The effect on plasma TG concentration is proportional to the baseline TG value and is commensurate with the ability of the statin to lower LDL-C

- Raise HDL-C to a small extent, the increase not dose related and reportedly greater in patients with low HDL-C

- Shown in randomized, controlled trials to increase long-term survival after heart transplantation

- Treatment begun at minimum dosage; plasma lipids and alanine transaminase (ALT) are measured at 6- to 8-week intervals; if necessary, dosage is increased stepwise

- Patients with very high pretreatment LDL-C may need combined therapy with a resin; statins may also be combined with caution with niacin (increased risk for myopathy or liver dysfunction) or with caution with a fibrate (increased risk for myopathy)

- A few patients have reversible creatine kinase elevations; rare myopathy (possible when combined with cyclosporine, fibrate, or perhaps niacin or erythromycin); minor elevations of serum transaminases, usually transient, can occur; prolongation of prothrombin time may occur when lovastatin given with coumarin

- Should not be used in women of childbearing potential unless contraception is fully satisfactory

- Absolute contraindication in active or chronic liver disease, or unexplained persistent elevations of serum transaminases; withhold if any acute or serious condition predisposing to the development of renal failure secondary to rhabdomyolysis

- Monitor liver enzymes before treatment and periodically thereafter, particularly if abnormal liver-function tests or substantial use of alcohol

Continued on next page

Statins—*Continued*

- Clinical trial evidence: significant reduction of clinical event rates in primary prevention (WOSCOPS, AFCAPS/TexCAPS) and secondary prevention (4S, CARE, LIPID), including CHD events (all events trials), stroke (CARE, LIPID), all-cause mortality (4S, LIPID); antiatherogenicity/decreased lesion progression (FATS, CCAIT, Post-CABG, REGRESS, LCAS, others)

DOSAGE

Administered in tablet form

- Atorvastatin   10–80 mg once daily, any time of day
- Cerivastatin   0.1–0.4 mg/day in the evening
- Fluvastatin   20–80 mg at bedtime
- Lovastatin   10–80 mg/day once nightly with the evening meal, or in divided doses
- Pravastatin   10–40 mg once daily, any time of day
- Simvastatin   5–80 mg in the evening

Table D.6-2. Effects of HMG-CoA Reductase Inhibitors on Major Lipid Fractions in Clinical Efficacy Studies at FDA-Approved Dosages

Agent	Disorder	Follow-up, wk	Dosage, mg	LDL-C	HDL-C	TG
Atorvastatin	1° HC	6	10 q.d.	-39	+6	-19
		6	20 q.d.	-43	+9	-26
		6	40 q.d.	-50	+6	-29
		6	80 q.d.	-60	+5	-37
Cerivastatin	1° HC	8	0.2 q.d.	-25	+9	-16*
		8	0.3 q.d.	-31	+8	-16*
		8	0.4 q.d.	-34	+7	-16*
Fluvastatin	Type IIa or IIb hyperlipidemia	9	20 q.p.m.	-22	Small but significant increases	Corresponding decreases
		4	40 q.p.m.	-24		
		4&8	40 b.i.d.	-35		
Lovastatin	Familial or nonfamilial HC	6	10 q.p.m	-21	+5	-10
		6	20 q.p.m.	-27	+6	+9
		6	10 b.i.d.	-28	+8	-7
		6	40 q.p.m.	-31	+5	-8
		6	20 b.i.d.	-32	+2	-6
		av 12&48	40 b.i.d.	-40	+10	-19
Pravastatin[†]	1° HC	8	10 q.p.m. @bed	-22	+7	-15
		8	20 q.p.m. @bed	-32	+2	-11
		8	40 q.p.m. @bed	-34	+12	-24
Simvastatin	1° HC	6	5 q.p.m.	-26	+10	-12*
		6	10 q.p.m.	-30	+12	-15*
		6	20 q.p.m.	-38	+8	-15*
		av 18&24	40 q.p.m.	-41	+9	-18*
		av 18&24	80 q.p.m.	-47	+8	-24*

Mean % Change from Baseline

Source: Data from *Physicians Desk Reference*, ed. 53. Oradell, NJ: Medical Economics Co., 1999, except data for cerivastatin (from May 1999 Professional Package Insert).

Note: @bed = at bedtime; b.i.d. = twice daily; HC = hypercholesterolemia; q.d. = daily; q.p.m. = each evening.

*Median % change.

[†]In 2000, time of dosing was changed to once daily, any time of day (see Table D.6-1).

Read in conjunction with manufacturers' product information sheets. In some countries, the dosage recommendations may vary; consult product labeling.

Table D.6-3. Bile-Acid Sequestrants (Resins)

Effective in lowering LDL-C, both in FH (at full dosage) and in other forms of hypercholesterolemia resistant to lifestyle changes (often in lower, more easily tolerated dosage)

- At the simplest level, these anion exchange resins nonspecifically bind bile acids (which are cholesterol rich) in the gut, increasing the bile salts' fecal excretion and interrupting their enterohepatic recirculation
- HDL-C increases slightly
- Because TG may increase, resins are not suitable in combined (mixed) hyperlipidemia unless a TG-lowering drug is also given; absolute contraindication in familial type III hyperlipidemia or TG >500 mg/dL (>5.6 mmol/L), relative contraindication TG >200 mg/dL (>2.3 mmol/L)
- Combination with a statin may be useful in severe hypercholesterolemia; resins may be combined with all other lipid-regulating drugs
- Little systemic toxicity; upper and lower GI complaints not uncommon, chiefly constipation and indigestion (absolute contraindication with history of severe constipation; use with great care in diabetic patients with GI autonomic neuropathy); can decrease absorption of other drugs (digitoxin, warfarin, thyroxine, thiazide diuretics, beta-blockers); can decrease absorption of folic acid and lipid-soluble vitamins
- Orange-flavored Colestid contains phenylalanine and should not be used in patients with phenylketonuria
- Patient should take other drugs 1–3 hours before or 4 hours after resin; bulking laxatives for constipation; folic acid and iron supplementation usual in pediatric patients
- Monitor complete blood count once yearly
- Clinical trial evidence: significant reduction of clinical CHD events in primary prevention (LRC-CPPT), antiatherogenicity/decreased lesion progression (FATS, STARS—also decreased CHD events in these small secondary-prevention trials)

DOSAGE

Administered as powders mixed with liquid or in tablet form (swallowed whole with water). Taken twice daily with meals, or daily at low dose

- Cholestyramine   4–24 g/day
- Colestipol   5–30 g/day

Read in conjunction with manufacturers' product information sheets. In some countries, the dosage recommendations may vary; consult product labeling.

Table D.6-4. Fibric-Acid Derivatives (Fibrates)

Particularly useful in patients with combined (mixed) hyperlipidemia or HTG; type IIb with elevated LDL-C, elevated TG, and low HDL-C; type III, IV, or V; type III is a prime indication for fibrates (marked reduction of lipoprotein remnant concentrations and xanthoma regression are the rule); well tolerated

- The most important clinical effects of fibrates are mediated through alterations in transcription of genes encoding for proteins that control lipoprotein metabolism and vascular inflammation (see also E.1.3)
- Reduce plasma TG effectively; increase HDL-C substantially
- May be used in mild to moderate hypercholesterolemia, in which LDL-C may be lowered. Effect on LDL-C variable, but LDL-C may increase if not initially elevated, especially if HTG is present. A substantial LDL-C increase may occur in a subset of nonresponders; marked LDL-C reduction may occur in a subset of responders
- May be combined with a resin, niacin, or (with caution) a statin (increased risk for myopathy)
- Transient transaminase increases not infrequent; can potentiate effects of oral anticoagulants; all rare—heartburn, nausea, diarrhea, gallstones, alopecia, muscle weakness with increased creatine kinase, loss of libido and potency. Absolute contraindication in hepatic or severe renal dysfunction (including primary biliary cirrhosis), preexisting gallbladder disease; avoid in diabetic nephropathy
- Monitor liver enzymes after initiation of therapy and at 4- to 6-month intervals thereafter
- Clinical trial evidence: significant reduction of clinical CHD event rates in primary prevention (Helsinki Heart Study) and secondary prevention (HIT); antiatherogenicity/decreased lesion progression (BECAIT, LOCAT)

DOSAGE

Administered in tablet (capsule) form with (especially in the case of gemfibrozil) a meal

- Bezafibrate   200 mg x 2 or 3 daily, or sustained-release form 400 mg daily
- Ciprofibrate   100 mg daily
- Fenofibrate   100 mg x 3 daily, or micronized form 200 mg x 1 daily (recommended U.S. starting dosage 67 mg/day)
- Gemfibrozil   600 mg x 2 daily (900–1,500 mg/day may be used)

Read in conjunction with manufacturers' product information sheets. In some countries, the dosage recommendations may vary; consult product labeling.

Table D.6-5. Nicotinic Acid (Niacin)

Appropriate in all Fredrickson phenotypes except type I

- The mechanisms are not well understood. Hypotheses include 1) inhibition of lipolysis in adipose tissue (decreased transport of nonesterified fatty acids to the liver could reduce hepatic VLDL production), 2) direct inhibition of hepatic synthesis or secretion of apo B–containing lipoproteins
- Effectively lowers both LDL-C and plasma TG and effectively increases HDL-C
- May be combined with a resin, fibrate, or statin (increased risk for myopathy or liver dysfunction when used with a statin)
- Side effects tend to limit compliance; flushing and GI symptoms are the most common problems; dry skin, pruritus, hepatotoxicity, hyperglycemia, hyperuricemia, or gout can also occur; both rare—acanthosis nigricans and retinal edema
- To minimize flushing: initial dose titration; take with meals and avoid taking with hot drinks, alcohol, or spicy food (low-fat snack with once-nightly Niaspan); as necessary, aspirin 30 minutes before administration (if aspirin not tolerated, ibuprofen may be substituted)
- Absolute contraindication in chronic liver disease; relative contraindication in type 2 diabetes, severe gout, or hyperuricemia; may potentiate effects of antihypertensive agents
- Follow liver enzymes, blood glucose, uric acid; check after each dose increase or if symptoms change, or at 3- to 6-month intervals if dose stable
- Clinical trial evidence: significant reduction of clinical CHD event rates in secondary prevention (Coronary Drug Project); antiatherogenicity/decreased lesion progression (CLAS, FATS)

DOSAGE

Available as tablets. Use sustained-release preparations with caution because of increased risk for hepatotoxicity

- Crystalline (immediate release) 1.5–6 g/day,* suggested with breakfast and dinner
- Extended release (Niaspan) 1–2 g at bedtime*
- Slow release 1–2 g/day,* suggested with breakfast and dinner

*Therapy with nicotinic acid must be initiated at low dosages, then titrated to desired response. Do not substitute slow- or extended-release formulations for equivalent dosages of crystalline nicotinic acid.

Read in conjunction with manufacturers' product information sheets. In some countries, the dosage recommendations may vary; consult product labeling.

Table D.6-6. Oral Estrogen-Replacement Therapy

May be considered to improve lipid profile in postmenopausal women

- Both estrogen and progesterone appear to influence lipoprotein metabolism at multiple regulatory points
- Decreases LDL-C moderately
- Increases HDL-C moderately
- May significantly increase TG, especially if patient has HTG
- Decision to use ERT must take into account menopausal symptoms and risks for CHD, osteoporosis, cancer, and thromboembolism (see Table B.3-1)
- Concomitant progestin administration in women who have not undergone hysterectomy, to reduce or eliminate increased risk for endometrial hyperplasia and endometrial cancer
- Because of an early increase in CHD events in a large, randomized prospective trial (HERS, using conjugated equine estrogens plus medroxyprogesterone acetate), it does not appear to be advisable to start estrogen–progestin therapy de novo in women with established CHD
- Appropriate monitoring for early evidence of endometrial cancer; also, adherence to standard recommendations for breast cancer screening prudent
- Clinical trial evidence: increased risk for nonfatal MI or CHD death during the first year of therapy (estrogen plus medroxyprogesterone), decreased risk during years 4 and 5, in the one published major trial (HERS, secondary prevention)

DOSAGE OF ESTROGENS

Administered in tablet form

- Conjugated estrogen   0.625 mg/day
- Micronized estradiol   2 mg/day

D.6.2 Possible Interactions

Table D.6-7. Selected Possible Drug and Food Interactions with Lipid-Regulating Agents

SEE LABELING INSTRUCTIONS OF MANUFACTURERS REGARDING SAFETY.

Drug Class	Interactive Agents	Manifestations of Drug Interactions
HMG-CoA reductase inhibitors (statins): atorvastatin, cerivastatin, fluvastatin, lovastatin, pravastatin, simvastatin	Immunosuppressant agents Fibric-acid derivatives Erythromycin Azole antifungals Cimetidine Grapefruit juice Methotrexate	Myopathy, rhabdomyolysis
	Nicotinic acid	Elevations in liver enzymes; possible muscle necrosis
	Coumarin	Prolongation of prothrombin time
	Bile-acid resins	Reduced statin absorption
Fibric-acid derivatives (fibrates): bezafibrate, ciprofibrate, fenofibrate, gemfibrozil*	Bile-acid resins Possibly antacids	Binding and decreased absorption of fibrate
	HMG-CoA reductase inhibitors Cyclosporine	Myopathy, rhabdomyolysis
	Warfarin-type anticoagulants	Increased anticoagulant activity

Continued on next page

*One published case report of potentiation of hypoglycemic action of glyburide with gemfibrozil (Ahmad *South Med J* 1991;84:102).

Table D.6-7—Continued

Drug Class	Interactive Agents	Manifestations of Drug Interactions
Nicotinic acid (niacin)	Aspirin (high dosage)	Increased concentration of nicotinic acid in the circulation
	Uricosuric agents (sulfinpyrazone)	Decreased efficacy of interactive agents
	Drugs that adversely affect hepatic structure or function	Hepatocellular necrosis
	HMG-CoA reductase inhibitors	Elevations in liver enzymes; possible muscle necrosis
	Antihypertensive agents	Possible potentiation of antihypertensive effects
Bile-acid sequestrants (resins): cholestyramine, colestipol	Thiazide diuretics Digitalis glycosides Beta-blockers Coumarin anticoagulants (warfarin) Thyroid hormones Gemfibrozil Oral hypoglycemic agents (sulfonylureas) Nonsteroidal antiinflammatory drugs	Binding and delayed or decreased absorption of interactive agents

Source: Adapted from Farmer JA, Gotto AM Jr. Antihyperlipidaemic agents: Drug interactions of clinical significance. *Drug Safety* 1994;11:301–309; used with permission.

D.6.3 Antihypertensive Drugs and Lipids

Table D.6-8. Effects of Selected Antihypertensive Drugs on Plasma Lipid Concentrations

Adverse lipid effects*

Beta-blockers, including

Nonselective beta-antagonists with no ISA, e.g., propranolol, timolol	Increase TG ($\uparrow\uparrow\uparrow$) Decrease HDL-C ($\downarrow$)
Highly selective beta-antagonists with no ISA, e.g., atenolol, metoprolol, betaxolol	Increase TG ($\uparrow\uparrow$) Decrease HDL-C ($\downarrow$)
Beta-antagonists with mild ISA, e.g., acebutolol	Increase TG ($\uparrow\uparrow$) Decrease HDL-C ($\downarrow$)

Diuretics,[†] including

Thiazides and thiazide-like diuretics	Increase TC, LDL-C, TG (modest and transient)
Loop diuretics, e.g., furosemide, ethacrynic acid	Increase TC and LDL-C (furosemide also lowers HDL-C)

Minimal or no lipid effects

Peripherally acting adrenergic inhibitors, e.g., reserpine, guanethidine, guanadrel

Direct vasodilators, e.g., hydralazine, minoxidil, diazoxide, sodium nitroprusside

Alpha- and beta-adrenergic blockers, e.g., labetalol

Angiotensin antagonists (ACE inhibitors), e.g., captopril, enalapril, lisinopril

Calcium antagonists, e.g., diltiazem, verapamil

Beneficial lipid effects

Beta-blockers, e.g., Pindolol (with partial ISA)	Does not modify TG May increase HDL-C
Centrally acting alpha agonists, e.g., methyldopa, clonidine, guanabenz, guanfacine	Decrease TC Decrease LDL-C
Alpha blockers, e.g., prazosin, terazosin, doxazosin	Decrease LDL-C Decrease VLDL-C Decrease TG Increase HDL-C

Note: ISA = intrinsic sympathomimetic activity.
Note: Hypertensive individuals have a higher than expected prevalence of hypercholesterolemia and vice versa. The two conditions increase CHD risk synergistically and should be treated aggressively when they coexist. Hypertension is linked with increases in plasma TG and decreases in HDL-C in the cardiovascular metabolic syndrome (see 1.3.6).
Note: See Table D.6-7 and manufacturers' labeling instructions regarding potential interactions of anti-hypertensive and lipid-regulating agents.
*Beta-blockers have been demonstrated in clinical trials to reduce total mortality, sudden death, and recurrent MI rates in MI survivors.
†The adverse lipid effects can be reduced or eliminated by cholesterol-lowering dietary modifications.

D.6.4 **S**UGGESTED **R**EADING

Adkins JC, Faulds D. Micronised fenofibrate: A review of its pharmacodynamic properties and clinical efficacy in the management of dyslipidaemia. *Drugs* 1997;54:615–633.

Brown WV. Niacin for lipid disorders: Indications, effectiveness, and safety. *Postgrad Med* 1995;98:185–189.

Crouse JR III. New developments in the use of niacin for treatment of hyperlipidemia: New considerations in the use of an old drug. *Coron Artery Dis* 1996;7:321–326.

Davignon J. Fibrates: A review of important issues and recent findings. *Can J Cardiol* 1994;10(suppl B):61B–71B.

Desager J-P, Horsmans Y. Clinical pharmacokinetics of 3-hydroxy-3-methylglutaryl-coenzyme A reductase inhibitors. *Clin Pharmacokinet* 1996;31:348–371.

Dujovne CA. New lipid lowering drugs and new effects of old drugs. *Curr Opin Lipidol* 1997;8:362–368.

Durrington P. Statins and fibrates in the management of diabetic dyslipidemia. *Diabetic Med* 1997;14:513–516.

Farmer JA, Gotto AM Jr. Antihyperlipidaemic agents: Drug interactions of clinical significance. *Drug Safety* 1994;11:301–309.

Garnett WR. Interactions with hydroxymethylglutaryl–coenzyme A reductase inhibitors. *Am J Health Syst Pharm* 1995;52:1639–1645.

LaRosa J. Review of clinical studies of bile acid sequestrants for lowering plasma lipid levels. *Cardiology* 1989;76(suppl 1):55–64.

Lea AP, McTavish D. Atorvastatin: A review of its pharmacology and therapeutic potential in the management of hyperlipidaemias. *Drugs* 1997;53:828–847.

Lennernäs H, Fager G. Pharmacodynamics and pharmacokinetics of the HMG-CoA reductase inhibitors: Similarities and differences. *Clin Pharmacokinet* 1997;32:403–425.

Miller DB, Spence JD. Clinical pharmacokinetics of fibric acid derivatives (fibrates). *Clin Pharmacokinet* 1998;14:156–162.

Shepherd J. Fibrates and statins in the treatment of hyperlipidaemia: An appraisal of their efficacy and safety. *Eur Heart J* 1995;16:5–13.

Spencer CM, Barradell LB. Gemfibrozil: A reappraisal of its pharmacological properties and place in the management of dyslipidaemia. *Drugs* 1996;51:982–1018.

Staels B, Vu-Dac N, Kosykh VA, et al. Fibrates downregulate apolipoprotein C-III expression independent of induction of peroxisomal acyl coenzyme A oxidase. A potential mechanism for the hypolipidemic action of fibrates. *J Clin Invest* 1995;95:705–712.

Tatò F, Vega GL, Grundy SM. Effects of crystalline nicotinic acid-induced hepatic dysfunction on serum low-density lipoprotein cholesterol and lecithin cholesteryl acyl transferase. *Am J Cardiol* 1998;81:805–807.

D.7 Other Treatment Options

Table D.7-1. LDL Apheresis and Other Treatment Options in Severe Refractory Hypercholesterolemia

LDL Apheresis

Description: Procedure for specifically removing apo B–containing lipoproteins from the blood. Most of the commonly employed systems have utilized immunoadsorption columns, dextran sulfate cellulose columns, and heparin precipitation.

Use: Approved by the U.S. Food and Drug Administration in 1996 for use in patients who despite diet and maximum tolerated drug therapy have:

- LDL-C >300 mg/dL (>7.8 mmol/L) when CHD is absent
- LDL-C >200 mg/dL (>5.2 mmol/L) when CHD is present

Usually performed in regional centers. A patient registry has been established to monitor clinical outcome and adverse effects.

Expected lipid effects of a single treatment: 120–150 mg/dL (3.0–4.0 mmol/L) decrease in LDL-C, 50–70% decrease in Lp[a], 50% decrease in VLDL-C and VLDL-TG, small reduction in HDL-C (dilutional effect)

Adverse events: Uncommon, including nausea/vomiting, flushing, and most commonly hypotension. Antihypertensive drugs need to be withheld immediately before LDL apheresis in patients at risk for hypotension. Hypotension can be severe in patients taking an ACE inhibitor.

Reported benefits: Stabilization of coronary atherosclerosis, functional improvement, reduced risk for restenosis after PTCA, reduced risk for graft vessel disease after heart transplantation, improved symptoms and stenoses in PVD

Use with statin therapy: Substantial additional LDL-C lowering achieved with high-dose atorvastatin (80 mg/day) and expanded-dose simvastatin (160 mg/day) in patients undergoing LDL apheresis for homozygous FH

Other Treatment Options

Used alone or combined with LDL apheresis: liver transplantation, portacaval shunt, plasmapheresis, partial ileal bypass surgery. Gene therapy appears to be a number of years away from routine clinical application.

D.8 Tactics for Enhancing Compliance with Lipid-Regulating Therapeutic Regimens

Table D.8-1. General Compliance Tactics

Tactic	Examples/Notes
Teach the patient to take the treatment regimen.	Instructions should be simple and concise but complete.
Help the patient identify ways to remember doses.	Tailor doses to daily habits. Send reminders.
Develop reinforcers of compliance.	Keep a chart of lipid responses. Provide continuing encouragement.
Anticipate common problems and teach the patient how to manage them.	Teach the patient how to minimize side effects.
Involve a family member or friend in the patient's therapy program.	Develop an advocate for the patient's welfare.
Establish a supportive relationship with the patient.	Listen carefully and respond in an open, non-judgmental manner.
Make compliance important by asking about it.	Develop an approach that is encouraging, not condemnatory.
Provide ongoing education and updates about the patient's illness and treatment.	Incorporate new data as the patient's level of understanding increases. Be on guard for mis-information the patient has received from the media, friends, or other sources.
Provide individualized services for patients who continue to avoid compliance.	Assess barriers: Physical—e.g., poor vision, forgetfulness Access—e.g., transportation, income, time Attitude—e.g., fatalism Therapy—e.g., complexity, side effects Social—e.g., family instability Faulty health perceptions—e.g., denial, looks to symptoms to prompt treatment

Source: Data from National Cholesterol Education Program. Second report of the Expert Panel on Detection, Evaluation, and Treatment of High Blood Cholesterol in Adults (Adult Treatment Panel II). *Circulation* 1994;89:1329–1445.

D.9 Cost Effectiveness of Lipid-Regulating Therapy

D.9.1 Overview

Cardiovascular disease imposes a massive economic burden for industrialized nations. It is estimated that the direct and indirect costs in 2000 for the United States alone will total U.S. $326.6 billion, including $118.2 billion related to CHD, $51.3 billion related to stroke, and $22.5 billion related to congestive heart failure (American Heart Association *2000 Heart and Stroke Statistical Update*). Economic analyses of lipid-regulating therapy are highly relevant. In many industrialized nations, CHD remains the leading killer, and plasma cholesterol elevation, a leading if not the leading risk contributor to CHD, is highly prevalent; in the United States, about 28% of adults are eligible for lipid-regulating therapy according to national (NCEP II) guidelines (Hoerger et al. *Am J Cardiol* 1998;82:61–65). As discussed in the Introduction, observational epidemiologic studies describe at least a 2–3% decrease in CHD risk for each 1% decrement in TC, and substantial morbidity and mortality reductions have been achieved in randomized trials of cholesterol-lowering drugs, including statistically significant decreases in all-cause death rates with HMG-CoA reductase inhibitor (statin) therapy in secondary prevention.

Available data suggest that population-wide lipid-regulating strategies emphasizing dietary modification are highly cost effective. Physician-prescribed cholesterol-lowering therapy can be highly cost effective when specific patient groups are targeted. As risk for CHD rises, whether through the accumulation of risk factors or increasing severity of risk factors, cost effectiveness improves. The most cost effective use of cholesterol-lowering drugs is in patients with established CHD, although cost effectiveness is also achieved in high-risk primary prevention. In addition, cost effectiveness tends to increase as more efficacious drugs, compared with less efficacious but equally expensive agents, are used. Nicotinic acid and statins have generally been described as more cost effective than other lipid-lowering agents. Cost effectiveness is of increased health policy concern with the statins because they have few side effects, which decreases concern about the risk:benefit ratio, and are at present relatively high cost.

How much a benefit is considered to be worth or what is considered to be affordable is largely a societal matter. The level of risk at which lipid-regulating drug therapy is recommended in national clinical practice guidelines appears to reflect the nation's type of healthcare system and the frequency of high-risk individuals. The relative difficulty of demonstrating cost effectiveness in the elderly when averted employment losses are considered and the greater cost effectiveness in men can represent, from a health policy perspective, discrimination against older persons and women.

D.9.2 Statin Therapy

In terms of U.S. dollars, health economists generally consider interventions to be highly cost effective if the cost per year of life saved (YLS) or quality-adjusted life years (QALY) is <$20,000, relatively cost effective if the cost/YLS or QALY is from $20,000 to $60,000, and expensive when cost/YLS or QALY exceeds $70,000. Estimates are that CABG for left main artery disease at $9,200/QALY (Weinstein and Stason *Circulation* 1982;66[III]:56–66) is highly cost effective, hydrochlorothiazide therapy for hypertension at $25,400/YLS (Edelson et al. *JAMA* 1990;263:407-413) is relatively cost effective, and CABG for mild angina and two-vessel disease at $72,900/QALY (Weinstein and Stason *Circulation* 1982;66[III]:56–66) is expensive (values updated to 1993 U.S. dollars by Kupersmith et al. *Prog Cardiovasc Dis* 1995;37:307–346). Data from prospective clinical trials now add to the evidence from economic simulation models that statin therapy is cost effective.

Cost-effectiveness analysis of the secondary-prevention **Scandinavian Simvastatin Survival Study** (4S), in which total mortality rate was highly significantly reduced by 30% with drug therapy (see 1.5.2), considered effects in patients aged 35, 59, and 70 years (the youngest, mean, and oldest ages at entry) and with TC of 213, 261, or 309 mg/dL (5.5, 6.7, or 8.0 mmol/L—the lowest, mean, and highest cholesterol concentrations at entry). Even when only direct costs were considered in 4S (1995 U.S. dollars), statin therapy ranged from highly cost effective ($3,800/YLS in 70-year-old men with TC of 309 mg/dL; $5,400/YLS in 59-year-old men with TC of 260 mg/dL; $10,500/YLS in 59-year-old women with TC of 260 mg/dL) to relatively cost effective ($27,400/YLS in 35-year-old women with TC of 213 mg/dL). When indirect costs, such as loss of productivity, were also considered, statin therapy was highly cost effective in all the 4S patients; results ranged from a savings in the youngest patients to a cost of $13,300 in 70-year-old women with TC of 213 mg/dL (Johannesson et al. *N Engl J Med* 1997;336:332–336).

In the primary-prevention **West of Scotland Coronary Prevention Study** (WOSCOPS), in which the CHD event rate was significantly reduced by 31% and the all-cause mortality rate was reduced by 22% (p = 0.51) with pravastatin therapy, cost/YLS when benefits were discounted ranged from ~$23,000 in the 40% of highest-risk men to ~$33,000 in all the middle-aged, hypercholesterolemic men studied (1996 U.S. dollars). Without discounting, the range was ~$9,000 to ~$13,000 (Caro et al. *BMJ* 1997;315:1577–1582). Hay et al. (*Circulation* 1997;96[suppl I]:I-184 [abstract]) estimated a base cost of $17,000/YLS upon projection of the WOSCOPS results to primary prevention in the United States, with therapy remaining cost effective across a wide range of risk factors and model assumptions. Thus, statin therapy as primary prevention in high-risk patients is at least relatively cost effective and may approach high cost effectiveness in highest-risk groups.

The economic value of statin therapy must also be viewed in terms of events averted, including significant reductions in MI, unstable angina, coronary revascularization procedures, hospitalization (reduced in terms of both number and length of stay), and, in some studies, stroke. The current low rate of use of lipid-lowering therapy, even in patients with CHD, can no longer be accepted.

D.9.3 Number Needed to Treat

Determination of number needed to treat (NNT), that is, the number of patients who need to be treated to achieve one benefit (prevent one event), is valuable because it takes into account overall risk, revealing benefit that is not apparent from relative risk reduction. NNT is calculated as 1 ÷ (treatment event rate - control event rate). As seen in Table 1.5-1, only 12 of the hypercholesterolemic, high-risk patients in **4S** needed to be treated for (on average) 5.4 years to prevent a major clinical coronary event, and only 30 needed to be treated to prevent a death from any cause. Prevention of a major clinical ischemic event in the secondary-prevention **Atorvastatin Versus Revascularization Treatments** (AVERT) trial required treatment of only 14 patients for 1.5 years. In the secondary-prevention **Veterans Affairs**

Cooperative Studies Program High-Density Lipoprotein Cholesterol Intervention Trial (HIT), 23 patients would need to be treated with gemfibrozil for 5 years to prevent one nonfatal MI or CHD death (Rubins et al. *N Engl J Med* 1999;341:410–418). Although prevention of a coronary event required treatment of larger numbers of the healthy patients in the primary-prevention statin trials, numbers are still small: an NNT of 45 in WOSCOPS (4.9 years) and 50 in the **Air Force/Texas Coronary Atherosclerosis Prevention Study** (AFCAPS/TexCAPS, 5.2 years). WOSCOPS investigators estimated that pravastatin treatment for 5 years of 1,000 middle-aged, hypercholesterolemic men with no history of MI will prevent 20 nonfatal MIs, 8 revascularization procedures, 7 CVD deaths, and 2 deaths from other causes (Shepherd et al. *N Engl J Med* 1995;333:1301–1307). They noted that these findings compare favorably with the results of the **Medical Research Council Trial** of the treatment of mild hypertension in middle-aged subjects, in which 5 years of treatment of 1,000 men aged 35–64 would result in 6 fewer strokes and 2 fewer CVD events than expected.

Meta-analysis of 23 trials of various lipid-regulating interventions in patients with CHD showed that only 16 patients with CHD need treatment for 5 years to prevent one major coronary event, and only 37 need treatment to prevent death from any cause (Rembold *J Fam Pract* 1996;42:577–586). Benefit was similar to that of other widely accepted secondary-prevention regimens (Table D.9-1). In the angiographic lipid-lowering trials, the NNT was 7 to prevent progression of coronary lesions, and 10 to induce lesion regression, across 2.5 years of treatment. Analysis of six primary-prevention trials (lasting on average 4.8 years and including WOSCOPS) showed that 53 patients need to be treated to prevent a nonfatal MI and 190 to prevent death from any cause (Rembold *J Fam Pract* 1996;42:577–586).

It is important to bear in mind that the greater the absolute risk reduction, the lower the NNT. For any given relative risk reduction, the benefit is greatest in the patients at highest risk. In the secondary-prevention **Cholesterol and Recurrent Events** (CARE) trial, for example, only 12 of the patients at increased risk because of the presence of diabetes mellitus (Goldberg et al. *Circulation* 1998;98:2513–2519) and 11 of the patients at increased risk because of greater age (65–75 years) (Lewis et al. *Ann Intern Med* 1998;129:681–689) needed to be treated for 5 years to prevent a major coronary event, in comparison with 33 of all CARE patients as calculated in Table 1.5-1. Sacks et al. (*Circulation* 1999;100[suppl I]:I-238–I-239 [abstract 1238]) in an assessment for the **Prospective Pravastatin Pooling Project** reported 5-year NNTs from pooled results of CARE and the **Long-term Intervention with Pravastatin in Ischemic Disease** (LIPID) trial of 11 for diabetic patients, 19 for nondiabetic patients, 13 for patients aged 65–75, and 23 for patients aged <55.

D.9.4 Improving Cost Effectiveness

How to maximize the cost effectiveness of lipid-lowering therapy is a crucial issue, in particular because recent trials such as **AFCAPS/TexCAPS** (Downs et al. *JAMA* 1998;279:1615–1622) have provided new evidence that CHD event benefit can also be achieved by statin therapy in patients with relatively low LDL-C concentrations and no known CHD at baseline (see 1.5.1). Improvements can be achieved in a number of ways, for example, by reductions in the cost of therapy or targeting patients most likely to have a cardiac event. Accurate prediction of patients most likely to suffer an infarction is difficult, however. The Second Joint Task Force of European and Other Societies on Coronary Prevention (*Eur Heart J* 1998;19:1434–1503) recommends targeting for lipid-regulating pharmacotherapy only those patients in whom the absolute CHD risk will exceed 20% over the next 10 years (or ~2%/year) or will exceed 20% if projected to age 60 (Figure A.2-1). In **WOSCOPS**, CHD rates exceeded 2%/year over 10 years if minor ECG abnormalities, smoking, HDL-C <43 mg/dL (<1.1 mmol/L), hypertension, or a family history of premature CHD was present (West of Scotland Coronary Prevention Group *Lancet* 1996;348:1339–1342). If the 40% of highest-risk WOSCOPS subjects (as opposed to all subjects) were targeted according to the suggested treatment threshold of 2%/year, the number needed to treat to prevent one event would decrease from ~40 to 22, greatly enhancing cost effectiveness (Ramsay et al. *Lancet* 1996;348:387–388; Jacobson et al. *Arch Intern Med* 1998;158:1977–1989).

Table D.9-1. Number Needed to Treat (NNT) Analysis Comparing Lipid-Regulating Therapy with Other Therapies

	No. of Trials	No. of Subjects	NNT	p Value
Secondary prevention, total mortality*				
Class I antiarrhythmics	11	4,336	22	<0.05
Anticoagulants	12	4,975	28	<0.05
Rehabilitation programs	23	5,022	31	<0.05
Beta-blockers	17	20,138	33	<0.05
Antidyslipidemics	23	18,452	37[†]	<0.05
Antiplatelet agents	9	13,917	37	<0.05
Dihydropyridines	6	13,114	625	NS
Treatment for acute MI, total mortality[‡]				
Thrombolysis	60	46,916	57	<0.05
Aspirin	5	19,077	62	<0.05
Anticoagulants	7	4,075	65	<0.05
Prophylactic lidocaine	15	8,745	95	NS
Beta-blockers	51	31,669	119	<0.05
Dihydropyridines	16	6,420	119	NS

Source: Rembold CM. Number-needed-to-treat analysis of the prevention of myocardial infarction and death by antidyslipidemic therapy. *J Fam Pract* 1996;42:577–586; used with permission.

Note: Value for lipid-regulating therapy was obtained by meta-analysis of 23 trials, including trials of lifestyle changes, drug therapy, and partial ileal bypass, reported from 1965 to 1995 and lasting a mean of 4.9 years. On average, active treatment resulted in an 18% reduction in TC. The only major clinical endpoints statin trial for which data were available was the Scandinavian Simvastatin Survival Study (4S).

*Total mortality was assumed to be similar to that observed in the control groups of all the antidyslipidemic trials (16% in 4.9 years).

†NNT = 16 to prevent nonfatal MI or CVD death.

‡Total mortality was assumed to be 7%.

E. PATHOPHYSIOLOGY

E.1 Summary of Lipid Metabolism

E.1.1 Plasma Lipoproteins

The major plasma lipoproteins, in order of increasing size and decreasing density, are high-density lipoprotein (HDL), low-density lipoprotein (LDL), intermediate-density lipoprotein (IDL), very low density lipoprotein (VLDL), and the chylomicron (Table E.1-1). Each is a sphere with a core of various amounts of triglyceride (TG) and cholesteryl ester, surrounded by a mono-layer of phospholipids, esterified (or "free") cholesterol, and specialized proteins called apolipoproteins. The apolipoproteins mediate lipoprotein catabolism by activating key lipolytic enzymes and associating with cellular receptors that remove lipoproteins from the plasma compartment. The structure and composition of the lipoproteins can be altered by various dyslipidemias (e.g., the small, dense LDL seen in association with hypertriglyceridemia [HTG]).

Chylomicrons are formed in the intestine following the breakdown and absorption of dietary fat; their major protein is apolipoprotein (apo) B-48. VLDL particles are assembled and secreted by the liver; their major protein is apo B-100. At the capillary endothelium, VLDL particles and chylomicrons are converted to IDL particles and chylomicron remnants, respectively, by the enzyme lipoprotein lipase (LPL), which is activated by apo C-II. Concurrently, the apo C proteins are transferred to HDL. LPL occurs at high concentrations in striated muscle and adipose tissue. The fatty acids freed by hydrolysis of chylomicron and VLDL TG are used as energy by muscle tissue or stored in adipose tissue to provide future energy.

Chylomicron remnants are removed by means of the LDL receptor–related protein. In the liver, IDL particles are converted to LDL by the action of hepatic lipase (HL), with the simultaneous transfer of apo E to other lipoproteins. LDL, whose sole major apolipoprotein is apo B-100, delivers cholesterol to peripheral cells (Figure E.1-1) for use in forming cell membranes and steroid hormones. The amount of cholesterol and fatty acids in mammalian cell membranes is controlled through a feedback system that is becoming better understood because of the recent discovery of a family of transcription-regulating proteins called sterol regulatory element–binding proteins (SREBPs). SREBPs are central to cholesterol homeostasis. Transcription is affected for a host of genes of lipid metabolism, including not only the LDL receptor but also 3-hydroxy-3-methylglutaryl coenzyme A (HMG-CoA) reductase, HMG-CoA synthase, farnesyl diphosphate synthase, acetyl CoA carboxylase, fatty acid synthase, and glycerol-3-phosphate acyltransferase. The coordinate regulation of so many genes associated with lipid metabolism is of great interest; its delineation may enable the design of new pharmacologic agents for the management of lipid disorders and atherosclerosis.

Plasma HDL particles are derived from the surface components that are released during the lipolysis of TG-rich lipoproteins and from cellular efflux of free cholesterol and phospholipids from peripheral tissue. These processes are mediated by lipases attached to the endothelium of peripheral and hepatic tissues and by ABC1, a plasma membrane protein found in peripheral tissue. The smallest HDL particles contain free cholesterol, phospholipids, and apolipoproteins. Through the acquisition of additional cholesterol and phospholipids, and the action of lecithin:cholesterol acyltransferase (LCAT), a small HDL particle increases in size and forms a core of cholesteryl ester. At least two plasma transfer proteins can exchange lipids between HDL, LDL, and VLDL particles; in the presence of HTG, efficient transfer of VLDL TG forms TG-rich LDL and HDL particles, which are converted to smaller species (e.g., small, dense LDL) by HL.

E.1.2 Lipoprotein Catabolism

Apo E is required for rapid hepatic removal of chylomicron remnants by means of the LDL receptor–related protein. More than 70% of LDL particles in healthy people are removed from plasma by means of the LDL (or B/E) receptor, which recognizes and binds LDL's apo B-100; most of these receptors are active in the liver. Hepatic uptake of either LDL particles or chylomicron remnants decreases their respective receptor activities and hepatic cholesterol biosynthesis.

A decrease in the number or activity of LDL receptors (e.g., with aging) leads to elevation of plasma cholesterol concentration. In the absence of receptor binding, LDL is not efficiently removed from plasma; further, without cholesterol uptake, cells continue to produce and secrete more cholesterol, for cholesterol biosynthesis is not down-regulated. A diet rich throughout life in saturated fat and cholesterol may lead to chronic suppression of LDL receptor activity. In homozygous familial hypercholesterolemia (FH), functional LDL receptors are absent, and total cholesterol concentrations reach 700–1,200 mg/dL (18–31 mmol/L).

LDL particles not removed by the LDL receptor are removed by other pathways; removal by cells of the reticuloendothelial system is collectively termed the scavenger cell pathway. The "scavenger receptor" of this route apparently recognizes only lipoproteins that have been chemically modified, for example, oxidized LDL. (See E.2.2.)

The mechanism of HDL catabolism is not clear. In humans HDL exists in two forms, HDL_2 and HDL_3, both of which contain apo A-I and apo A-II as their major apolipoproteins. Turnover data in humans are not unequivocal because they are based on exchangeable labels. Data from other species suggest that the larger species, HDL_2, is a precursor of HDL_3. In HTG subjects, the HDL_2, which is TG rich, is a substrate for HL (as noted above), which converts it to smaller HDL, presumably HDL_3. HDL_3 is the longest-lived lipoprotein (3–5 days) and one could argue that it is removed by nonspecific endocytosis. On the other hand, there is some evidence that HDL associates with cell surface receptors (e.g., liver, adrenals) that affect the translocation of HDL lipids. The murine class B, type I scavenger receptor (SR-BI) is the first molecularly well-defined cell surface HDL receptor to be described. (The human CD36 and LIMPII analogous FI [CLA-1] receptor shows high sequence homology with SR-BI.) A facilitator of both lipid influx and efflux in HDL, it mediates the selective removal of HDL cholesteryl ester by adrenal gland and liver (Figure E.1-2). Its expression is coordinately regulated with steroidogenesis in several sites. Interestingly, adenovirus-mediated hepatic overexpression of SR-BI in mice results in the virtual disappearance of plasma HDL and increased biliary cholesterol.

E.1.3 Insulin and Lipid Metabolism

Insulin plays a normal coordinating role in postprandial metabolism, and insulin resistance is associated with a cluster of metabolic alterations, including elevation of plasma TG and lowering of HDL-C, that are risk factors for atherosclerosis (Figure E.1-3, and see 1.3.6). It has been suggested that insulin resistance may affect lipid metabolism as much as it affects glucose metabolism. Significant advances have been made recently toward understanding the molecular events that regulate glucose and lipid homeostasis, notably through the identification of peroxisome proliferator–activated receptors (PPARs), nuclear receptors that are activated by fatty acids and their derivatives. The (antihyperlipidemic) fibrate and (antihyperglycemic) thiazolidinedione drugs, both of which have potent TG-lowering activity, have been identified as synthetic ligands for PPAR-α and PPAR-γ, respectively. Through PPAR-α mediation, fibrates decrease hepatic apo C-III mRNA levels and protein production and selectively induce LPL mRNA levels and activity in the liver. In addition, PPAR-α mediates fibrate action on HDL-C concentrations by means of transcriptional induction of synthesis of apo A-I and apo A-II. Thiazolidinediones, on the other hand, act chiefly on adipose tissue, with no effect in the liver. PPAR-α appears to have a modulatory role in the pathogenesis of several age-related disorders, including dyslipidemia, insulin resistance, and chronic inflammation, that predispose to atherothrombotic disease.

E.1.4 Biosynthesis of Cholesterol

The biosynthesis of cholesterol has been elucidated in considerable detail. The rate-limiting intermediate step in its derivation from acetate is the conversion of HMG-CoA to mevalonic acid by HMG-CoA reductase. It is this key step that is inhibited by the class of drugs termed HMG-CoA reductase inhibitors, or statins. The liver and intestine are the major sources of endogenously derived cholesterol. Generally, the body can manufacture all the cholesterol it needs. Cholesterol is needed for cell membrane biogenesis and the production of steroid hormones and bile salts. It is a key molecule in embryonic development.

E.1.5 Lipoproteins and Atherogenesis

The pathogenesis of atherosclerosis is reviewed in E.2. Pathogenically typical atherosclerosis is generated by diet-induced hypercholesterolemia in experimental models, and lipid-laden foam cells and advanced lesions with lipid-rich cores have been well documented in animals and human subjects in which LDL receptors are decreased or absent.

Derangements in lipid metabolism that are associated with elevated

LDL-C usually lead to premature atherosclerosis. Findings of molecular genetics, cell biology, animal studies, observational epidemiologic studies, and clinical trials all suggest that elevated LDL-C is involved in atherogenesis. However, the evidence that native LDL itself is an atherogenic lipoprotein is not as compelling, and there is particular interest in the role of oxidatively modified lipoproteins in the formation of the foam cells that characterize early atherosclerosis.

The inverse correlation between plasma HDL-C and premature atherosclerotic disease does not necessarily support HDL as an anti-atherogenic lipoprotein because low HDL-C is frequently associated with HTG, insulin resistance, low plasma LPL, and small, dense LDL, any one of which may be more closely linked to the mechanism for atherosclerosis. "HDL cardioprotection" has been hypothesized to result from postulated reverse cholesterol transport (Figure E.1-2). It has also been postulated that a protective effect of HDL could be direct, for example, through inhibition of smooth muscle cell proliferation or interference with macrophage uptake of oxidized LDL.

There is also clinical interest in lipoprotein[a] (Lp[a]), which is assembled from an LDL particle and a large, hydrophilic glycoprotein termed apo [a], which bears little resemblance to the other apolipoproteins. Research interest has arisen not only because of a positive epidemiologic association between plasma Lp[a] concentration and risk for CHD, but also because of the striking structural homology between apo [a] and plasminogen. It has been suggested that much of the atherogenic potential of Lp[a] derives from its interference in normal pathways of thrombolysis. Currently, no drugs exist that specifically lower Lp[a]. Nicotinic acid, LDL apheresis, and pharmacologic dosages of estrogenic hormones may lower Lp[a] to a degree to allow evaluation of clinical response. Some MI survivors exhibit fairly high concentrations of Lp[a] (e.g., >70 mg/dL) in the absence of well-established CHD risk factors. It may be appropriate to set an LDL-C target even lower than 100 mg/dL (2.6 mmol/L) in these patients (e.g., 80 mg/dL, or 2.1 mmol/L) because limited data have indicated that Lp[a] concentration may cease to be a risk factor when LDL-C concentrations are low enough. In general, an Lp[a] concentration >30 mg/dL is considered elevated.

Table E.1-1. Classification and Properties of Major Human Plasma Lipoproteins

Lipoprotein Class	Buoyant Density, kg/L	Flotation Rate, Sf, at 26°C and at a Background Density of 1.063 kg/L	1.20 kg/L	Mean Particle Mass (10^6 Da)	Electrophoretic Mobility	Major Apolipoprotein Content	Mean Diameter, nm
Chylomicron	<0.95	<400	—	1,000	Origin	B-48, C, E	100–1,000
Very low density lipoprotein (VLDL)	0.95–1.006	20–400	—	4.5–100	α_2 (pre-β)	B-100, C, E	30–70
Intermediate-density lipoprotein (IDL)	1.006–1.019	12–20	—	4.0	α_2–β	B-100, E	25
Low-density lipoprotein (LDL)	1.019–1.063	0–12	—	3.0	β	B-100	20
High-density lipoprotein (HDL) Subfraction 2	1.063–1.125		0–3.5	0.4	α_1	A-I, A-II, C	10
Subfraction 3	1.125–1.210		3.5–9	0.2	α_1	A-II, A-I, C	8

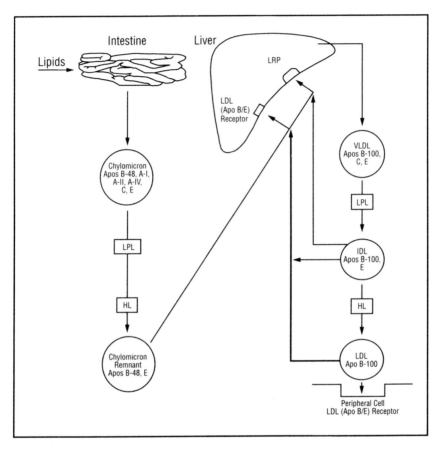

Figure E.1-1. Chylomicron, very low density lipoprotein (VLDL), and low-density lipoprotein (LDL) metabolism. Apo = apolipoprotein; HL = hepatic lipase; IDL = intermediate-density lipoprotein; LPL = lipoprotein lipase; LRP = LDL receptor–related protein.

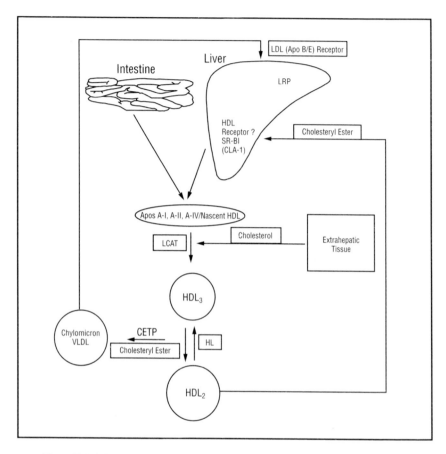

Figure E.1-2. Model of reverse cholesterol transport. The identification of a high-density lipoprotein (HDL) receptor—CLA-1 (human CD36 and LIMPII analogous F1 receptor)—in the liver suggests a mechanism of delivery of cholesteryl ester to the liver that differs from the receptor-mediated uptake of low-density lipoprotein (LDL). Apo = apolipoprotein; CETP = cholesteryl ester transfer protein; HL = hepatic lipase; LCAT = lecithin:cholesterol acyltransferase; LRP = LDL receptor–related protein; SR-BI = class B, type I scavenger receptor; VLDL = very low density lipoprotein.

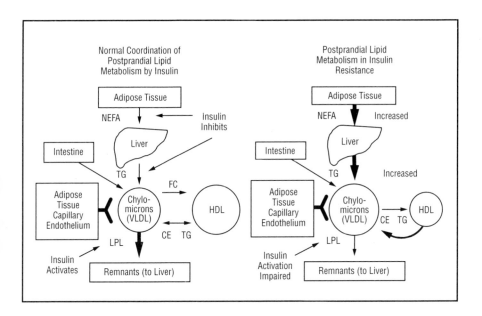

Figure E.1-3. Insulin resistance and the cardiovascular metabolic syndrome.
Under normal circumstances, lipid metabolism is regulated by insulin, particularly in the postprandial period. Insulin inhibits the release of nonesterified fatty acids (NEFA) from adipose tissue and the secretion of very low density lipoproteins (VLDL) by the liver. Insulin also stimulates lipoprotein lipase (LPL), an enzyme that is localized in capillaries and that hydrolyzes VLDL and chylomicron triglyceride (TG). All these effects lead to a reduction in circulating TG-rich particles (VLDL and chylomicrons). In insulin resistance, the release of NEFA from adipose tissue and of VLDL from the liver is increased and the breakdown of these particles by LPL is reduced. This leads to an increase in circulating TG-rich remnant lipoprotein particles, which are thought to be particularly atherogenic. Secondarily, there is a reduction in high-density lipoprotein (HDL) cholesterol concentration because of increased exchange of VLDL and chylomicron TG for cholesteryl ester (CE) in HDL by the action of cholesteryl ester transfer protein. FC = free (nonesterified) cholesterol.

Modified from the International Task Force for Prevention of Coronary Heart Disease. Coronary heart disease: Reducing the risk. The scientific background for primary and secondary prevention of coronary heart disease. A worldwide view. *Nutr Metab Cardiovasc Dis* 1998;8:205–271; used with permission.

E.2 Evolution and Stabilization of Atherosclerotic Lesions

E.2.1 Classification of Lesions

Atherosclerosis is classified as a systemic disorder of the arteries, but it typically occurs at specific, so-called lesion-prone sites, including sites near arterial branches and bifurcations as well as regions of vessel narrowing and curvature. Mechanical forces such as fluid shear stress play a role throughout the evolution of the disease, including plaque progression and rupture. Disease occurs principally in the elastic arteries (aorta, carotid, and iliac) and some of the large and medium-sized muscular arteries (coronary and popliteal).

Although the exact mechanisms of atherosclerosis remain a subject of debate, the disease has been well described morphologically. The American Heart Association classification, in which an evolutionary sequence is implicit, describes six histologic types. Lesion types I–III are silent precursors of advanced lesions. Fatty streaks (type II), which typically first appear in the coronary arteries around puberty, contain macrophage foam cells as their chief component. Type III (intermediate) lesions and the first atheroma-type lesions tend to be found in young adults. Type IV lesions, or atheromas, are characterized by a lipid core, separated from the endothelium largely by smooth muscle cells and macrophages. Type V lesions are distinguished by the formation of prominent new fibrous connective tissue; type Va contains a lipid core whereas type Vc does not, and in type Vb the lipid core and other parts of the lesion are calcified. Type IV and type V lesions may develop fissures, hematoma, and/or thrombus to become type VI (complicated) lesions. These complications account for most ischemic events. In western populations, advanced lesions containing thrombi or their remnants are frequent from the fourth decade of life on. A key determinant of the rates at which atherosclerosis develops in different populations is lifestyle.

E.2.2 Lesion Formation and Progression

The leading hypothesis of atherogenesis is that lesions arise as an immune/inflammatory, or healing, response of the intima to injury. With chronic minimal injury, the endothelium may become dysfunctional yet remain structurally intact; abnormal vasoconstriction is now increasingly recognized as one of the earliest manifestations of endothelial dysfunction. Among factors associated with endothelial dysfunction/injury are hypercholesterolemia, active and passive cigarette smoking, hypertension, a high-fat diet, advanced glycosylated end products in diabetes mellitus, obesity, insulin resistance, and physical inactivity. Complex changes in activated endothelium, such as changes in vascular permeability and alterations in expression of endothelial cell adhesion receptors, lead to monocyte recruitment into the vessel wall, one of the pivotal initiating events in atherosclerosis.

Within the intima, monocytes are converted into macrophages, which can internalize large amounts of lipid to become foam cells. The source of the lipid is plasma lipoproteins, in particular LDL. How the lipoproteins come to be trapped in the artery wall, instead of returning to the plasma compartment, has not been well delineated, although proteoglycans are believed to play a major role. LDL must be modified for macrophage uptake. Oxidative modification is the best studied of candidate modifications. Higher susceptibility to lipid peroxidation is seen in LDL from subjects with risk factors such as CHD, diabetes mellitus, or smoking, and in small, dense LDL. In the artery wall LDL oxidation is believed to occur in two stages, wherein minimal modification precedes and promotes monocyte recruitment, and full oxidation occurs after monocytes/macrophages contribute their great oxidative capacity. The protein (apo B-100) of LDL becomes more negatively charged during the latter process, leading to loss of recognition by the LDL (apo B/E) receptor and a shift to recognition by macrophage scavenger receptors and/or the oxLDL receptor. Unlike LDL receptor–mediated uptake, this uptake is not down-regulated. Macrophages that die within the intima instead of exiting with their lipid load can contribute to the formation of the lipid core of an atherosclerotic lesion.

In addition to providing a morphologic basis for foam cells (smooth muscle cells account for a minority of foam cells), monocytes/macrophages can release a variety of substances (e.g., growth factors, cytokines, procoagulants, cytotoxic substances) that may have far-reaching consequences for atherosclerosis proliferation, vascular remodeling, and plaque destabilization. Similarly, about 20 potentially proatherothrombotic properties of oxidized LDL have been described beyond its role in the genesis of foam cells, although in vivo relevance has been validated for only a few.

Measurement of a variety of molecules such as oxidation products and adhesion molecules may serve to indicate the presence of vascular endothelial dysfunction or inflammation, or of early atherosclerosis, perhaps without duplication of other risk assessments. There is a high degree of interest in C-reactive protein (CRP). In the future, measurement of this marker of vascular inflammation may be useful to refine risk assessment in intermediate-risk patients and might enable improved targeting of therapy.

Fibrous plaque development is characterized by smooth muscle cell migration and proliferation, which are promoted by a variety of growth-regulatory molecules (e.g., tumor necrosis factor α, interleukin 1, platelet-derived growth factor) that are up-regulated in atherosclerotic lesions. Typically, a fibrous cap forms over a lesion with a lipid core. Its connective tissue matrix is produced by the smooth muscle cells; numerous cytokines control a balance of collagen synthesis and degradation. Caps are often thinnest at their shoulder regions, where macrophage and metalloproteinase activity is high and disruption most frequently occurs.

How plaques progress is highly variable and poorly understood. Coronary lesion progression is usually sudden and unpredictable. Plaque disruption is common, and a large proportion of plaques that cause high-grade stenosis result from previous disruption. Plaque growth is usually clinically silent.

E.2.3 Onset of Acute Coronary Syndromes

Although continued plaque growth and abnormal coronary vasomotor tonal responses in atherosclerotic arteries can also be causative, most clinical symptoms of CHD, including angina, MI, and death, occur because of the development of a thrombus large enough to protrude into the vessel lumen and acutely decrease blood flow. Acute thrombosis usually results from plaque rupture or from erosion of a fibrous plaque. According to necropsy and atherectomy studies, the plaques most likely to rupture are those with a large lipid core, a thin cap, high macrophage density, and reduced smooth muscle cell content (Figure E.2-1). The macrophages are activated and probably responsible for the destruction of the connective tissue of the cap through metalloproteinases such as stromelysin 1. Other factors associated with disruption may include juxtaposed regions of contrasting composition, lumen irregularities and asymmetry, and endothelial dysfunction. The likelihood of a clinical ischemic event relates to the number of vulnerable lesions present. Even one strategically located rupture-prone lesion, however, can lead to death. Lesions rich in lipid appear to be not only more vulnerable to rupture but also more thrombogenic when the lipid is exposed to circulating blood. (Key points of the management of thrombogenic risk factors are shown in Table E.2-1.)

There is no readily apparent relation between plaque composition and plaque size or the degree of stenosis. Most clinical ischemic events result from lesions causing only mild or moderate stenosis because those lesions are much more numerous in the arterial tree than lesions causing severe obstruction. Indeed, because of vascular remodeling, some advanced lesions do not encroach on the lumen at all and are angiographically invisible. Moreover, because hemodynamically insignificant narrowing does not stimulate the development of collateral vessels, the sequelae of sudden complete occlusion at such a site can be more severe.

E.2.4 Lesion Regression and Stabilization

Until the 1980s, when angiographically monitored clinical trials showed that intensive lipid modification could retard coronary lesion progression and in a small subset of patients lead to regression, the general view was that human atherosclerosis was irreversible, unaffected by any influence less drastic than wartime starvation. There is an apparent discrepancy in such trials, however, in that despite only small absolute improvements in coronary stenosis (1–2% according to a multitrial analysis by Brown et al. [*Circulation* 1993;87:1781–1791]), reductions in CHD events with intervention have been large. Rossouw (*Am J Cardiol* 1995;76:86C–92C) found a 47% reduction in cardiovascular events in pooled results of angiographic trials. That analysis accords with the significant reductions in risk for coronary events, in the range of 23% to 37%, at 5–6 years in clinical endpoint trials (WOSCOPS, AFCAPS/TexCAPS, 4S, CARE, and LIPID) of HMG-CoA reductase inhibitors, or statins (see 1.5). Given this angiographic–clinical paradox and the unexpected finding that most clinical ischemic events arise from lesions that cause only mild or moderate angiographic stenosis but are unstable and prone to rupture, the concept of lesion stabilization to reduce risk for disability and death has emerged. The term is a loose one, referring to beneficial effects on plaque biology unrelated to major changes in stenosis and encompassing reduced propensity to plaque rupture/thrombosis and improvement in abnormal vasomotor function (Table E.2-2).

Thus, it has been hypothesized that lipid-regulating therapy may achieve its clinical benefit at least in part through mechanisms other than effects on stenosis. Among mechanisms for which evidence is available for the statins are effects on vascular reactivity, rheologic/thrombotic effects, modulation of immune function, and reduced oxidation potential. Many of these effects have been seen within 3 months of the beginning of therapy. Interestingly, benefit in coronary event rates has been reported from statin clinical endpoint trials within 6–12 months. Williams et al. (*J Am Coll Cardiol* 1998;31:684–691) found plaque characteristics more consistent with lesion stability in cynomolgus monkeys treated for 2 years with very high dosage pravastatin than in untreated monkeys. Fibrate effects include well-described effects on hemostatic variables. In at least 12 studies, lipid lowering with a statin, resin, or LDL apheresis very quickly (e.g., within 2–4 weeks) improved endothelium-dependent vasomotor function in patients with and without CHD and with marked or borderline hypercholesterolemia. It may be that anything that substantially lowers LDL (including oxidized LDL) may make arteries respond more like healthy arteries. Among other interventions that may have similar endothelial effects are smoking cessation, blood pressure reduction, regular exercise, antioxidant therapy (vitamins C and E or probucol), estrogen replacement, and ACE inhibition. Distinguishing lipid and nonlipid effects is not straightforward: for example, oxidized LDL is proinflammatory, and lipoproteins modulate the expression and/or function of a variety of rheologic, fibrinolytic, and thrombotic factors (e.g., LDL promotes platelet activation and tissue factor expression).

A high proportion of acute clinical coronary ischemic events appear to be triggered by external factors such as emotional stress or morning waking. Proposed mechanisms include plaque disruption and vasoconstriction. Trigger reduction may also help prevent or delay clinical events. Target triggers include smoking and, in the physically unfit, unaccustomed vigorous exertion. Beta-blockers, ACE inhibitors, and heart rate–reducing calcium antagonists may also modify triggering mechanisms.

Table E.2-1. Management of Thrombogenic Risk Factors

Lifestyle changes

- Smoking cessation
- Reduction of overweight
- Low intake of saturated fat and increased intake of omega-6* and omega-3 polyunsaturated fatty acids (seed oils and oily fish)
- Increased intake of foods providing B vitamins and folate

Drug therapy

- The favorable effect of antiplatelet drugs on cardiovascular risk is maximal immediately after the ischemic event, and lasts for about 36 months.
- The effect of antiplatelet drugs is maximal when they are combined with smoking cessation, a cholesterol-lowering diet, and control of arterial hypertension.
- The recommended dosage of aspirin is 75–160 mg/day, taken after food.
- For prevention of thrombosis in coronary bypass grafts or after PTCA, aspirin may be given alone or in combination with dipyridamole. Ticlopidine (250 mg b.i.d.) may be used as an alternative to this combination. Ticlopidine use should be monitored by white cell counts because of the risk for neutropenia.
- Data from the large Clopidogrel versus Aspirin in Patients at Risk of Ischaemic Events (CAPRIE) trial showed that clopidogrel (75 mg/day) is more effective than aspirin (325 mg/day) in patients suffering from thrombotic complications of atherosclerosis (CAPRIE Steering Committee *Lancet* 1996;348:1329–1339).
- Hemorrhagic stroke and GI bleeding were reported in early studies of oral anticoagulants, antiplatelet drugs, and thrombolytic agents. In more recent studies, these have been less common. Risk for GI bleeding is lowest when the smallest doses of aspirin are used.
- Warfarin dosage is adjusted to maintain the international normalized ratio (INR) between 2.0 and 3.5.
- Hypersensitivity is a side effect of all antithrombosis drugs and precludes their use in some patients.
- Like smoking cessation and weight reduction, use of fibric-acid derivatives lowers plasma fibrinogen.

Source: Data from The International Task Force for Prevention of Coronary Heart Disease. Coronary heart disease: Reducing the risk. The scientific background for primary and secondary prevention of coronary heart disease. A worldwide view. *Nutr Metab Cardiovasc Dis* 1998;8:205–271; used with permission. Available at www.chd-taskforce.com.

ILIB note: Data are not available to support safety of increased intake of linoleic acid.

Table E.2-2. Potential Approaches to Prevention of Adverse Consequences of Coronary Atherosclerosis

• Prevention of atherosclerosis and its progression and facilitation of regression

• Plaque stabilization
    Reduced vulnerability to rupture
        ↓ Lipid core or modification of its composition
        ↓ Macrophage density or matrix-degrading activity
        ↑ SMC density and matrix synthesis
    Elimination of extrinsic triggers to plaque rupture
    Reduced plaque thrombogenicity
        ↓ Lipid core
        ↓ Macrophage density and tissue factor content/activity
    Improved endothelial function
        Restoration of normal vasodilator function
        Reduced prothrombotic phenotype
        Reduced proinflammatory phenotype
        In each case:
            ↓ Lipid core
            ↓ Lipid concentrations
            ↓ Lipid peroxidation

• Improved systemic thrombotic–thrombolytic equilibrium

• Promotion of collateral recruitment

Source: Shah PK. Pathophysiology of plaque rupture and the concept of plaque stabilization. *Cardiol Clin* 1996;14:17–29; used with permission.

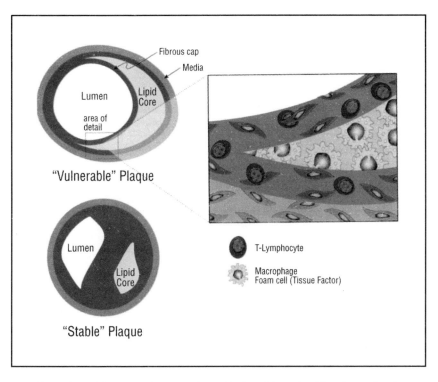

Figure E.2-1. Diagrammatic comparison of vulnerable and stable atherosclerotic plaques. A vulnerable plaque typically has a substantial lipid core and a thin fibrous cap that separates macrophages (bearing tissue factor) from the blood. In a stable plaque, in contrast, a relatively thick fibrous cap protects the lipid from contact with the blood. Because plaque growth is initially outward, the lumen is often well preserved when a vulnerable plaque is present, whereas clinical data suggest that stable plaques more often cause angiographic luminal narrowing. From Libby P. Molecular bases of the acute coronary syndromes. *Circulation* 1995;91:2844–2850; used with permission.

F. ADDITIONAL RISK ISSUES
F.1 Risk for Stroke

Table F.1-1. Risk Factors for First Ischemic Stroke

Modifiable, Value Established	Potentially Modifiable	Unmodifiable
Well-documented Hypertension Cardiac disease: Atrial fibrillation, infective endocarditis, mitral stenosis, recent large MI Cigarette smoking Sickle cell disease TIAs Asymptomatic carotid stenosis	*Well-documented* Diabetes mellitus Hyperhomocysteinemia LV hypertrophy *Less well documented* Elevated blood lipids Cardiac disease: cardiomyopathy, segmental wall motion abnormalities, nonbacterial endocarditis, mitral annular calcification, mitral valve prolapse, valve strands, spontaneous echocardiographic contrast, aortic stenosis, patent foramen ovale, atrial septal aneurysm Use of oral contraceptives Consumption of alcohol Use of illicit drugs (most commonly, cocaine; also, heroin, amphetamines, LSD, PCP, others) Physical inactivity Obesity Elevated hematocrit Dietary factors Hyperinsulinemia and insulin resistance Acute triggers (e.g., stress) Migraine Hypercoagulability and inflammation: fibrin formation and fibrinolysis, elevated fibrinogen, anticardiolipin antibodies, genetic and acquired causes Subclinical disease: intimal–medial thickness, aortic atheroma, ankle–brachial blood pressure ratio, infarctlike lesions on magnetic resonance imaging Socioeconomic features	*Well-documented* Age Male sex* Hereditary/familial factors Race/ethnicity Geographic location *Less well documented* Season and climate

Source: Adapted from Sacco RL, Benjamin EJ, Broderick JP, et al. Stroke risk factors. American Heart Association Prevention Conference IV: Prevention and Rehabilitation of Stroke. *Circulation* 1997;96:701–707. ©1997 American Heart Association, Inc. Used with permission.
Note: The probability of ischemic stroke is increased severalfold by the presence of multiple risk factors.
Note: **Stroke recurrence:** Most studies characterized risk factors for initial stroke, whereas longitudinal studies often emphasized survival rather than recurrence. Some but not all studies found no effect of hypertension and cardiac disease.
Note: Risk factors for **intracerebral hemorrhage** include age, male sex, race/ethnicity, hypertension, LV hypertrophy, prior stroke, heavy use of alcohol, use of cocaine, anticoagulation and thrombolytic therapy, and, in the elderly, amyloid angiopathy. Incidence of **subarachnoid hemorrhage** increases only moderately with age, and age-adjusted risk is higher in women. Other risk factors for subarachnoid hemorrhage include race/ethnicity, family history, hypertension, cigarette smoking, and certain diseases (e.g., polycystic kidney disease, coarctation of the aorta, Marfan syndrome).
*Each year in the United States, however, more women than men die of stroke because they tend to live longer than men.

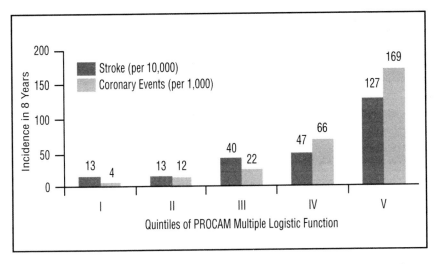

Figure F.1-1. Observed incidences of stroke and coronary events in quintiles of estimated coronary risk (multiple logistic function) among men aged 40–65 years in PROCAM (Münster Heart Study). There were 258 coronary and 48 cerebrovascular events in 8 years among 4,849 men recruited from 1979 to 1985. An important result of PROCAM is that the risk algorithm for coronary events (fatal or nonfatal MI or sudden cardiac death) also identifies men at high risk for fatal or nonfatal stroke. Variables used in the algorithm, all independent predictors of coronary events, are age, LDL-C, HDL-C, SBP, TG, cigarette smoking, diabetes mellitus, and a family history of MI. The rate of increase across the quintiles of the PROCAM algorithm is similar for observed coronary and cerebrovascular events. Modified in format from PROCAM Slide Kit, downloadable at www.chd-taskforce.com; used with permission. (See also Figure 2.4-1 and Table 3-1 regarding PROCAM prediction of coronary events.)

Table F.1-2. Recommendations from the National Stroke Association (United States) for Prevention of a First Stroke

Good evidence for intervention

1. Treatment of hypertension, including isolated systolic hypertension in the elderly
2. Warfarin use in post-MI patients with atrial fibrillation, decreased LV ejection fraction, or LV thrombus
3. HMG-CoA reductase inhibitor (statin) use in post-MI patients with normal to high cholesterol concentrations (see 1.5.2)
4. Warfarin use in patients with atrial fibrillation and specific risk factors
5. Carotid endarterectomy for patients with asymptomatic stenosis ≥60% but <100% when local surgical morbidity and mortality risk is <3%

Support from observational studies

6. Smoking cessation
7. Control of alcohol use (proposed J-shaped relation between alcohol use and ischemic stroke rate)
8. Increased physical activity
9. Diet,* including decreased sodium intake; consumption of adequate amounts of fruits and vegetables; consumption of folate, vitamin B6, and vitamin B12 in amounts adequate to prevent elevated plasma homocysteine

Additionally

10. Measures to improve compliance with therapies

Source: Data from Gorelick PB, Sacco RL, Smith DB, et al. Prevention of a first stroke. A review of guidelines and a multidisciplinary consensus statement from the National Stroke Association. *JAMA* 1999;281:1112–1120.

ILIB note: The National Stroke Association advisory board did not find evidence substantial enough to allow the conclusion that antiplatelet agents are useful in preventing a first stroke after MI. Aspirin therapy is recommended for the prevention of subsequent MI, however. The International Task Force/International Atherosclerosis Society notes that aspirin (at least 325 mg/day) reduces risk for stroke in atrial fibrillation by 10–20%, and that in secondary prevention of ischemic stroke aspirin and ticlopidine are of value (*Nutr Metab Cardiovasc Dis* 1998;8:205–271).

ILIB note: The International Task Force/International Atherosclerosis Society also recommends prevention of the development of diabetes mellitus (whether aggressive glycemic control in diabetes will lower stroke risk is uncertain) and treatment of obesity, LV hypertrophy, valve disease, and patent foramen ovale (*Nutr Metab Cardiovasc Dis* 1998;8:205–271).

*The American Heart Association notes that fish, green tea, and milk in increased amounts were protective against stroke, whereas diets high in fat and cholesterol could be deleterious (Sacco et al. *Circulation* 1997;96:701–707).

G. ADDITIONAL RESOURCES

G.1 Online Resources

Table G.1-1. Selected World Wide Web Resources

Organization	Address
American Academy of Pediatrics	www.aap.org
American Cancer Society	www.cancer.org
American Diabetes Association	www.diabetes.org
American Dietetic Association	www.eatright.org
American Heart Association	www.americanheart.org
International Task Force for Prevention of Coronary Heart Disease	www.chd-taskforce.com*
The Living Heart	www.livingheart.com†
National Lipid Education Council	www.lipidhealth.org
U.S. Agency for Health Care Policy and Research	www.ahcpr.gov‡
U.S. Centers for Disease Control and Prevention	www.cdc.gov§
U.S. National Heart, Lung, and Blood Institute	www.nhlbi.nih.gov
World Health Organization	www.who.int

Note: Many of the selected sites contain links to other national and international sites of interest.

*Includes the PROCAM interactive CHD risk calculator as well as clinical recommendations and scientific background for the management of multiple CHD risk factors.

†Provides information for patient education.

‡Includes smoking cessation guide for primary-care physicians developed by a panel convened by the AHCPR of the U.S. Public Health Service working with the U.S. Centers for Disease Control and Prevention.

§Includes the U.S. Surgeon General's reports on physical activity and smoking.

INDEX

ABC1 protein, E.1.1

absolute risk, higher: in diabetic patients, B.1.2; in the elderly, B.4.1, B.4.2.1; and improved cost effectiveness, 1.5.1, D.9.3, D.9.4; in Joint Task Force guidelines, Figure A.2-1. *See also* risk calculators, CHD

ACE inhibitors, E.2.4, Tables A.2-1, D.6-8

AFCAPS/TexCAPS (Air Force/Texas Coronary Atherosclerosis Prevention Study), 1.5.1, Tables 1.5-1, 1.5-2, Figure 1.5-1; cost effectiveness, D.9.3; and low HDL-C, 1.3.2; pharmacoeconomic issues raised by, D.9.4; results in the elderly, B.4.2.1, Table B.4-1; results in women, B.3.2.1

aging, Table 2.4-1; delayed risk for CHD in women, B.3.1; elderly, B.4.2

alcohol: cardioprotective effect, D.2.2.4; effects in women, B.3.2; maximum intake, Tables 2.8-1, B.1-2; in Mediterranean diet, D.2.2.3, Table D.2-2; restriction in hypertriglyceridemia, Tables A.1-5, D.1-1; risks, 2.4, D.2.2.4

algorithm, treatment, for dyslipidemia: ILIB, diabetic adult, Chart B.1-1; ILIB, general adult, Charts 2-1, 2-2; Joint Task Force, adult, Figure A.2-1; NCEP, adult, A.1; NCEP, pediatric, Tables B.2-1, B.2-5

alpha-glucosidase inhibitors, Table B.1-2

angina pectoris: in the elderly, B.4.3; onset of, E.2.3; reduction of, Table 1.5-2; in women, B.3.1

angiographic trials of lipid-regulating therapy, 1.6, Table 1.6-1; and HDL-C, 1.3.2; and triglyceride-rich lipoproteins, 1.3.3; in women, B.3.2.1

antihypertensive drugs: in diabetic patients, Table B.1-2; in the elderly, B.4.4; lipid effects, Table D.6-8

antioxidants, D.2.2.9, E.2.4

apheresis, LDL, Tables 2.6-1, D.7-1; and endothelial function, E.2.4

apo [a], E.1.5

apo B, as clinical CHD predictor, Table C.1-1

apo B-48, E.1.1, Figure E.1-1

apo B-100, E.1.1, Figure E.1-1; familial defective, Table 2.6-1

apo C-II deficiency, 1.3.3, Table 2.6-1

apo E, E.1.1, E.1.2, Figure E.1-1; E2/2 phenotype/genotype, Tables 2.6-1, C.1-2 apolipoproteins, E.1.1, Table E.1-1

Asian–Pacific CHD Risk Factor Collaborative Group, 1.1

Asia, traditional diet/lifestyle in, 1.3.1

aspirin: as antiplatelet agent, Tables A.2-1, E.2-1; given with niacin, Tables D.6-5, D.6-7

atherogenesis, E.2; beginnings in childhood, B.2.1; and triglyceride-rich lipoproteins, 1.3.3

atherosclerosis: experimental, 1.3.1; histologic types, E.2.1; initiation and progression, E.2.2; risk in Fredrickson phenotypes, Tables 2.2-2, 2.6-1; rupture-prone lesions, E.2.3, Table E.2-2, Figure E.2-1

atorvastatin: dosage, Table D.6-1; in FH, 3.11, Tables 2.6-1, D.7-1; major lipid effects, Table D.6-2. *See also* AVERT; IDEAL; MIRACL; TNT

AVERT (Atorvastatin Versus Revascularization Treatments) trial, 1.5.2, Tables 1.5-1, 1.5-2; cost effectiveness, D.9.3

BECAIT (Bezafibrate Coronary Atherosclerosis Intervention Trial), 1.3.3, 1.6, Table 1.6-1

beta-blockers, E.2.4, Tables A.2-1, D.6-8

bezafibrate: dosage, Table D.6-4. *See also* BECAIT; BIP; SENDCAP

bile-acid sequestrants: in combination-drug lipid-lowering therapy, Table D.6-3; dosage, Table D.6-3; major lipid effects, Tables 2.9-3, D.6-3; mechanisms, Table D.6-3; side effects, Table D.6-3; use in the elderly, Table B.4-2; use in pediatric patients, 3.14, B.2.4, Table B.2-5. *See also* cholestyramine; colestipol

BIP (Bezafibrate Infarction Prevention) trial, 1.3.3

blood pressure: in the elderly, B.4.2, B.4.4; goal in diabetic adults, Table B.1-2; 95th percentile in youths, Table B.2-3. *See also* hypertension

body mass index, Tables D.3-1, D.3-3

bruits, vascular, Tables 2.3-1, C.2-1

bupropion, Table D.5-1; in diabetic patients, Table B.1-2

bypass, partial ileal: for refractory severe hypercholesterolemia, Table D.7-1; results in POSCH, B.3.2.1, Table 1.6-1

CABG. *See* revascularization, coronary

calories, nutrition, Table 2.8-1; estimating daily need for, Table D.2-1; restriction of, Table D.3-4

CAPRIE (Clopidogrel versus Aspirin in Patients at Risk of Ischemic Events) trial, Table E.2-1

carbohydrate, Table 2.8-1; for diabetic patients, Table B.1-2; and plasma triglyceride, 1.4, D.2.2.1; and reduction of chylomicronemia, Table 2.6-1

cardiovascular metabolic syndrome, 1.3.6, 3.3, Figure E.1-3; aspects in youths, B.2.4; and diabetes mellitus, B.1.2; hypertriglyceridemia as marker for, 1.3.3, Table C.2-1

CARE (Cholesterol and Recurrent Events) trial, 1.5.2, Tables 1.5-1, 1.5-2; cost effectiveness, D.9.3; results in diabetic patients, B.1.3.1, Table B.1-3; results in the elderly, B.4.2.1, Table B.4-1; results in women, B.3.2.1

CCAIT (Canadian Coronary Atherosclerosis Intervention Trial), Table 1.6-1; results in women, B.3.2.1

cerivastatin: dosage, Table D.6-1; major lipid effects, Table D.6-2

CHD mortality rates: in diabetic patients, B.1.2; dietary trials, 1.4; effects of cholesterol-lowering drug therapy on, 1.5.1, 1.5.2; and estrogen-replacement therapy, B.3.4; international trends, 1.1; total plasma cholesterol as risk factor for, 1.3.1

CHD symptoms: in the elderly, B.4.3; in women, B.3.1

Chicago Heart Association Study, 1.2

cholesterol: biosynthesis, E.1.4; delivery to peripheral cells, E.1.1, Figure E.1-1; total plasma, as CHD risk predictor, 1.3.1. *See also* cutpoints, lipid

cholesterol, dietary: contribution to atherosclerosis, E.1.2, E.1.4; effect of reducing, Table D.1-1; maximum intake, Tables 2.8-1, A.1-7

Cholesterol Treatment Trialists' Collaboration, B.4.2.1

cholestyramine: combined with a statin, 3.11; dosage, Table D.6-3; in pediatric patients, 3.14. *See also* LRC-CPPT; STARS

chylomicron, 2.2.2, E.1.1, Table E.1-1, Figures E.1-1, E.1-2

chylomicronemia, 1.3.3, Tables 2.2-2, 2.6-1, A.1-5; in pediatric patients, B.2.4; recognition of, Table C.1-1; use of fish oil in, D.6.1

ciprofibrate: dosage, Table D.6-4

CLA-1 receptor, E.1.2, Figure E.1-2

Clinical Quality Improvement Network, 1.1

clofibrate. *See* Coronary Drug Project; Stockholm Ischemic Heart Disease Secondary Prevention Study

clopidogrel, Table E.2-1

colestipol: dosage, Table D.6-3. *See also* FATS

combined hyperlipidemia, 3.9, 3.13, Tables 2.2-2, 2.6-1, 2.9-2, C.2-1

compliance, enhancing, Table D.8-1; in the elderly, B.4.4.2. *See also* undertreatment

computed tomography, technetium-99m sestamibi (MIBI) single-photon emission, 3.11

contraception, oral, 2.4, B.3.2

conversion of units of measure for cholesterol and triglyceride, Table C.1-2, inside back cover

Copenhagen Male Study, 1.3.3, 1.3.6

corneal arcus, Tables 2.6-1, C.2-1

Coronary Drug Project, 1.5.2

coronary heart disease. *See* CHD

cost effectiveness, D.9; number needed to treat, D.9.3, Tables 1.5-1, D.9-1; of statin therapy, 1.5.1, D.9.2

CURVES trial, 3.10

CRP (C-reactive protein), E.2.2

cutpoints, lipid: in diabetic patients, Tables B.1-4, B.1-5, Chart B.1-1; ILIB adult, 2.2.1, Table 2.2-1, Table 2.9-1, Charts 2-1, 2-2; Joint Task Force, Figure A.2-1; NCEP adult, Tables A.1-2, A.1-4, A.1-5; NCEP pediatric, B.2.3, Table B.2-4, Table B.2-5.

DCCT (Diabetes Control and Complications Trial), B.1.2

diabetes mellitus, B.1, Chart B.1-1; case study, 3.4; cost effectiveness of lipid-lowering therapy, D.9.3; diagnosis of, B.1.1, Table B.1-1; dyslipidemia in pediatric patients, B.2.5; type 1, B.1.5; and type III hyperlipidemia, Table 2.6-1; in women, B.1.2, B.1.3, B.3.2

diet, cholesterol-lowering: 2.8, Table 2.8-1; clinical trials, 1.4, Table 1.6-1; in diabetes mellitus, Table B.1-2; implementation, D.2; in youths, B.2.4, Table A.1-7

diet, Mediterranean, D.2.2.3, Table D.2-2

Diet, Step I, Table A.1-7; in youths, B.2.4

Diet, Step II, Table A.1-7; in the elderly, B.4.4.1; in pediatric patients, B.2.4

drug therapy, lipid-regulating: angiographically monitored trials, 1.6; available agents, D.6.1; clinical endpoint trials, 1.5.1, 1.5.2; in diabetes mellitus, B.1.4.2, Table B.1-6; effects on major plasma lipids, Table 2.9-3; in the elderly, B.4.4.2, Table B.4-2; initiation of, ILIB, 2.9; initiation of, NCEP, Tables A.1-4, A.1-5; interactions with drugs and food, potential, Table D.6-7; in pediatric patients, B.2.4, Table B.2-5; selection of agents, 2.9.2; underutilization, 1.1; in women, B.3.2.1

dysbetalipoproteinemia. *See* type III hyperlipidemia

egg consumption, D.2.1, Table 2.8-1

elderly, B.4; case study, 3.7; cost effectiveness of lipid-lowering therapy, D.9.3; decreased LDL receptor activity in, E.1.2

endothelial function, 1.7, B.3.4, E.2.4, Table E.2-2

energy intake. *See* calories, nutrition

estrogen replacement therapy, B.3.4, Tables B.3-1, D.6-6

EUROASPIRE (European Action on Secondary Prevention through Intervention to Reduce Events), 1.1

exercise: benefits, 1.3.6, Table D.1-1; in diabetes mellitus, Table B.1-2; classifications, Table D.4-3; in the elderly, B.4.4; lipid effects, Table D.1-1; recommendations, Tables D.4-1, D.4-2; in weight control, Table D.3-4; in youths, B.2.2

FAME (Fluvastatin Assessment of Morbidity/Mortality in the Elderly), 3.7

family history: obtaining, Table C.3-1; as risk factor, 2.6, Tables 2.3-1, 2.4-1; unobtainable, in youths, Table B.2-1

fat, grams of: equivalence to energy intake, Table D.2-1

FATS (Familial Atherosclerosis Treatment Study), Table 1.6-1

FCH (familial combined hyperlipidemia), 3.13, Tables 2.6-1, A.1-5, C.2-1; and cardiovascular metabolic syndrome, 1.3.6; in children, B.2.3; and diabetes mellitus, B.1.3

fenofibrate: dosage, Table D.6-4

FH (familial hypercholesterolemia): heterozygous, 2.6, 3.11, 3.14, B.2.3, B.3.2.1, Tables 2.6-1, C.2-1, D.7-1; homozygous, E.1.2, Tables 2.6-1, D.7-1

fiber, soluble, D.2.2.6

fibric-acid derivatives: case studies, 3.3, 3.8, 3.9; in combination-drug lipid-lowering therapy, Table D.6-4; dosage, Table D.6-4; major lipid effects, Tables 2.9-3, D.6-4; mechanisms, E.1.3, E.2.4, Table D.6-4; side effects, Table D.6-4; use in the elderly, B.4.4.2, Table B.4-2. *See also* bezafibrate; gemfibrozil

fibrinogen, 1.3.6, 2.4, Table D.1-1

fish consumption, D.2.2.5, Tables 2.8-1, D.1-1, E.2-1

fish oil, 3.8, D.2.2.5, D.6.1

fluvastatin: dosage, Table D.6-1; major lipid effects, Table D.6-2. *See also* FAME; LCAS

folic acid supplementation: and homocysteine, D.2.2.8; with resin use, Table D.6-3

food selection for cholesterol lowering, Table 2.8-1, D.2.1

4S. *See* Scandinavian Simvastatin Survival Study

Framingham Study: risk calculator, 1.2, Table 3-1; risk factor decreases, 1.1; TC:HDL-C ratio, 1.3.4, B.3.2

Fredrickson phenotypes, 2.2.2, Tables 2.2-2, 2.6-1

Friedewald formula, Table C.1-2

gemfibrozil: dosage, Table D.6-4. *See also* Helsinki Heart Study; HIT; LOCAT

gene therapy for hypercholesterolemia, Table D.7-1

glucose tolerance, impaired: CARE findings, B.1.3.1; case studies, 3.2, 3.3, 3.8; in the cardiovascular metabolic syndrome, 1.3.6; defined, B.1.1; lifestyle changes for, Table D.1-1; and risk for macrovascular disease, B.1.2

glycemic control, B.1.2, B.1.4.1, Table B.1-2

goals, lipid, Tables 2.2-1, 2.7-1; in diabetes mellitus, Table B.1-2. *See also* algorithm, treatment, for dyslipidemia

HDL (high-density lipoprotein), E.1.1, E.1.2, Table E.1-1, Figure E.1-2

HDL cholesterol: case studies of patients with low, 3.2–3.4, 3.9; case study of patient with high, 3.5; and CHD risk, 1.3.2, B.3.2, E.1.5; cutpoints in adults, ILIB, Table 2.2-1; cutpoints in diabetic adults, Table B.1-5, Chart B.1-1; drug therapy for, 2.9.1, Tables 2.9-1, 2.9-3, A.1-6; familial low, 1.3.2, 2.5, Table 2.6-1; high, 2.5, Table A.1-3; lifestyle changes to raise, D.2.2.2, Table A.1-6; low, causes of secondary, 1.3.2, 2.5; low, in diabetic patients, B.1.3, B.1.4.2; in youths, Table B.2-4

Hegsted equation, Table 2.8-1

Helsinki Heart Study, 1.5.1; results in diabetic patients, B.1.3.1, Table B.1-3

hepatic lipase, E.1.1, Figures E.1-1, E.1-2

hepatosplenomegaly, Tables 2.6-1, C.2-1

HERS (Heart and Estrogen–Progestin Replacement Study), B.3.4

HIT (Veterans Affairs Cooperative Studies Program High-Density Lipoprotein Cholesterol Intervention Trial), 1.3.2; cost effectiveness, D.9.3; results in diabetic patients, B.1.3.1, Table B.1-3; results in the elderly, B.4.2.1, Table B.4-1; and stroke reduction, 1.5.2

HMG-CoA (3-hydroxy-3-methylglutaryl coenzyme A) reductase, E.1.4

HMG-CoA reductase inhibitors: in combination-drug lipid-lowering therapy, Table D.6-1; dosage, Table D.6-1; major lipid effects, Tables 2.9-3, D.6-1, D.6-2; mechanisms, Table D.6-1, E.1.4, E.2.4; side effects, Table D.6-1; and stroke reduction, 1.5.2, Table F.1-2; use in diabetic patients, B.1.3.1, B.1.4.2, Tables B.1-3, B.1-6; use in the elderly, B.4.4.2, Table B.4-2; use with estrogen replacement, B.3.4; use in pediatric patients, 3.14, B.2.4, Table B.2-5; use posttransplantation, Table D.6-1. *See also* atorvastatin; cerivastatin; fluvastatin; lovastatin; pravastatin; simvastatin

homocysteine, 2.4, D.2.2.8

hyperapobetalipoproteinemia (hyper–apo B), 1.3.6, Table 2.6-1 hypercholesterolemia: and atherogenesis, E.1.5; case studies of patients with, 3.1, 3.5–3.7, 3.9–14; causes of secondary, Tables 2.5-1, C.2-1; choice of drug therapy, Table 2.9-2; common presentations, Table C.2-1; polygenic, Table 2.6-1; treatment of refractory severe, Table D.7-1. *See also* cholesterol; FH

hyperinsulinemia, 1.3.6, 2.4

hypertension, 1.3.6, Tables 2.4-1, A.1-3; control in diabetes mellitus, B.1.2

hypertriglyceridemia: case studies of patients with, 3.3, 3.4, 3.8, 3.9, 3.13; causes of secondary, Table 2.5-1; choice of drug therapy, Table 2.9-2; common presentations, Table C.2-1; in diabetes mellitus, B.1.3; dietary treatment of, D.2.2.1; familial, B.1.3, Table 2.6-1; and Friedewald formula, Table C.1-2; management of, in adults, 2.5–2.11, Table A.1-5; management of, in pediatric patients, B.2.4. *See also* chylomicronemia; triglyceride, fasting plasma

hypertrophy, left ventricular, B.4.2

hypothyroidism: in diabetic patients, B.1.4; in the elderly, B.4.3

IDEAL (Incremental Decrease in Endpoints through Aggressive Lipid Lowering) trial, 1.5.2

IDL (intermediate-density lipoprotein), E.1.1, Tables C.1-1, E.1-1, Figure E.1-1

insulin: and atherogenesis, B.1.2; exogenous, B.1.4.1; and lipid metabolism, E.1.3; resistance, 1.3.6, 2.4

insulin resistance syndrome. *See* cardiovascular metabolic syndrome

insulin secretagogues, Table B.1-2

insulin sensitizers, Table B.1-2

Internet resources, Table G.1-1

Johns Hopkins Precursors Study, 1.3.1

Kumamoto Study, B.1.2

laboratory standardization, Table C.1-1

LCAS (Lipoprotein and Coronary Atherosclerosis Study), 1.3.2, Table 1.6-1

LCAT (lecithin:cholesterol acyltransferase), E.1.1, Figure E.1-2

LDL (low-density lipoprotein): oxidation, B.1.3, E.1.2, E.2.2; small, dense, 1.3.6, 2.4, 3.3, B.1.3, E.1.5, Table C.1-1

LDL cholesterol: and CHD risk, 1.3.1; estimation of, Table C.1-2. *See also* cutpoints, lipid

LDL (apo B/E) receptor, E.1.2, E.2.2, Figures E.1-1, E.1-2

lifestyle: assessment of need for changes in, 2.7; lipid goals, Table 2.7-1; lipid effects of modified, Table D.1-1; westernization of, 1.1, 1.3.1, B.1.1, B.2.2

lipemia retinalis, Table 2.6-1

LIPID (Long-term Intervention with Pravastatin in Ischemic Disease) trial, 1.5.2, Tables 1.5-1, 1.5-2; cost effectiveness, D.9.3; results in diabetic patients, B.1.3.1, Table B.1-3; results in the elderly, B.4.2.1, Table B.4-1; results in women, B.3.2.1

lipid metabolism, E.1

LOCAT (Lopid Coronary Angiography Trial), 1.3.2, 1.6, Table 1.6-1

Los Angeles Veterans Administration Study, 1.4

lovastatin: dosage, Table D.6-1; major lipid effects, Table D.6-2. *See also* AFCAPS/TexCAPS; CCAIT; FATS; Post-CABG

Lp[a] (lipoprotein[a]), 2.4, E.1.5; elevated, E.1.5; and estrogen replacement, B.3.4; and Friedewald formula, Table C.1-2

LPL (lipoprotein lipase), E.1.1, E.1.3, Figure E.1-1; deficiency, 1.3.3, Table 2.6-1

LRC-CPPT (Lipid Research Clinics Coronary Primary Prevention Trial), 1.5.1; and HDL-C, 1.3.2

LRP (LDL receptor–related protein), E.1.1, Figures E.1-1, E.1-2

Lyon Diet Heart Study, D.2.2.3

MEDFICTS Dietary Assessment Questionnaire, D.2.1

Medical Research Council/British Heart Foundation Heart Protection Study, 3.7

Medical Research Council Trial of treatment of mild hypertension, D.9.3

meta-analysis: angiographic trials, E.2.4; cost effectiveness, D.9.3; non-statin secondary-prevention trials, 1.5.2; plasma cholesterol and CHD mortality, 1.3.1, 1.5.2, 3.10; plasma cholesterol and total mortality, 1.5.2, 3.10; plasma triglyceride as CHD predictor, 1.3.3; statin therapy and stroke, 1.5.2

metformin, B.1.2, B.1.4.1, Table B.1-2

microalbuminuria, 1.3.6, 2.4, Table B.1-4

MIRACL (Myocardial Ischemia Reduction with Aggressive Cholesterol Lowering) trial, 1.5.2

monounsaturated fatty acids, D.2.1, D.2.2.3, Tables 2.8-1, D.2-2

mortality, total: and multiple risk factors, 1.2; and plasma cholesterol, 1.3.1; reduction with lipid-regulating therapy, 1.3.1, 1.5.1, 1.5.2

MRFIT (Multiple Risk Factor Intervention Trial): CVD risk in diabetes mellitus, B.1.2; CHD risk from multiple factors, 1.2

multiple risk factors: assessment for, 2.4, Table 2.3-1; synergistic effects of, 1.2; in Helsinki Heart Study, 1.5.1. *See also* risk calculators, CHD

Münster Heart Study: estimate of overall risk for CHD, Table 2.4-2, Figure 2.4-1; LDL-C:HDL-C ratio as CHD predictor, 1.3.4; lipid triad as CHD predictor, 1.3.5; plasma triglyceride as CHD predictor, 1.3.3, Figure 1.3-1; PROCAM risk calculator, 1.2, Figure F.1-1, Table 3-1; stroke prediction, Figure F.1-1; TC:HDL-C ratio as CHD predictor, 1.3.4, Figure 1.3-2

Muscatine Study, B.2.2

myocardial infarction: measurement of lipids after, Table C.1-1; pathophysiology of onset, E.2.3. *See also* CHD symptoms

neuropathy, gastrointestinal autonomic, Table B.1-6

NHANES (National Health and Nutrition Examination Survey): effects of multiple risk factors, 1.2, Figure 1.2-1; findings on undertreatment, 1.1; mean cholesterol in U.S. adults, 3.12

niacin. *See* nicotinic acid

nicotine replacement therapy, Table D.5-1

nicotinic acid: in combination-drug lipid-lowering therapy, Table D.6-5; dosage, Table D.6-5; major lipid effects, Table D.6-5; mechanisms, Table D.6-5; side effects, Table D.6-5; use in diabetic patients, B.1.4.2, Table B.1-6; use in the elderly, Table B.4-2; use in pediatric patients, B.2.4, Table B.2-5. *See also* Coronary Drug Project; FATS; Stockholm Ischemic Heart Disease Secondary Prevention Study

Ni–Hon–San Study, 1.3.1

non-HDL-C, Table C.1-1

North Karelia Project, 1.1

number needed to treat. *See* cost effectiveness

Nurses' Health Study, and estrogen replacement, B.3.4

obesity: case studies, 3.2, 3.8; classification, Table D.3-1; as contributor to cardiovascular metabolic syndrome, 1.3.6; as major risk factor for CHD, Table 2.4-1; risk in Helsinki Heart Study, 1.5.1. *See also* weight control

olive oil, D.2.2.3, Table 2.8-1

omega-3 fatty acids. *See* fish consumption; fish oil

omega-6 fatty acids, Tables 2.8-1, E.2-1

Oslo Diet–Heart Study, 1.4

overall risk for CHD, estimating, 2.4. *See also* risk calculators, CHD

overweight. *See* obesity

PAI-1 (plasminogen activator inhibitor 1), 1.3.6, 2.4

pancreatitis, 3.8, B.1.4, Tables 2.6-1, A.1-5

paradox, angiographic–clinical, E.2.4

PDAY (Pathobiological Determinants of Atherosclerosis in Youth) study, B.2.1

pediatric cardiovascular health schedule, Table B.2-2

pediatric risk assessment and management, B.2; case study, 3.14

peripheral pulses, Tables 2.3-1, C.2-1

physical activity. *See* exercise

plant stanols/sterols, D.2.2.10

pleiotropic effects, 1.5.2, 2.9.1, D.6.1, E.2.4

polyunsaturated fatty acids, Table 2.8-1. *See also* fish consumption; fish oil; omega-6 fatty acids

POSCH (Program on the Surgical Control of the Hyperlipidemias), Table 1.6-1; results in women, B.3.2.1

Post-CABG (Post Coronary Artery Bypass Graft) trial, 1.6, 3.9, Table 1.6-1; results in the elderly, B.4.2.1; results in women, B.3.2.1

PPARs (peroxisome proliferator–activated receptors), E.1.3, Table B.1-2

pravastatin: dosage, Table D.6-1; major lipid effects, Table D.6-2. *See also* CARE; LIPID; Prospective Pravastatin Pooling Project; PROSPER; REGRESS; WOSCOPS

pregnancy, dyslipidemia in, B.3.3, Table C.1-1

primary dyslipidemias, 2.6, Table C.2-1; in children, B.2.3

primary prevention of CHD: importance of, 1.1; lipid-lowering drug trials, 1.5.1. *See also* cutpoints, lipid; risk calculators, CHD

PROCAM (Prospective Cardiovascular Münster) study. See Münster Heart Study

progestin, B.3.4, Tables B.3-1, D.6-6

progression, atherosclerotic lesion. *See* angiographic trials of lipid-regulating therapy; atherosclerosis; ultrasound, B-mode

Project Heartbeat!, B.2.3

Prospective Pravastatin Pooling Project, 1.5.2; cost effectiveness, D.9.3

PROSPER (Prospective Study of Pravastatin in the Elderly at Risk), 3.7

proteinuria, Table B.1-4

PTCA. *See* revascularization, coronary

raloxifene, B.3.4

ratio, LDL-C:HDL-C: cutpoints in adults, ILIB, Table 2.2-1; as risk predictor, 1.3.4

ratio, TC:HDL-C: cutpoints in adults, ILIB, Table 2.2-1; as risk predictor, 1.3.4, Figure 1.3-2; in women, B.3.2

ratio, waist:hip, Table 2.3-1

REGRESS (Regression Growth Evaluation Statin Study), Table 1.6-1

regression, atherosclerotic lesion, E.2.4, Table E.2-2. *See also* angiographic trials of lipid-regulating therapy; ultrasound, B-mode

rehabilitation, cardiac, B.3.1, Table D.4-1. *See also* exercise

resins. *See* bile-acid sequestrants

revascularization, coronary: reduction with lipid-lowering therapy, 1.5.1, 1.5.2, Tables 1.5-1, 1.5-2

reverse cholesterol transport, E.1.5, Figure E.1-2

risk calculators, CHD, 1.2, Table 3-1

risk factors for CHD, major: ILIB, Table 2.4-1; NCEP, Table A.1-3

sampling, blood, Table C.1-1

saturated fatty acids, 1.4, E.1.2, E.1.4, Tables 2.8-1, D.1-1, D.2-1

Scandinavian Simvastatin Survival Study (4S), 1.5.2, Tables 1.5-1, 1.5-2; cost effectiveness, D.9.2; results in diabetic patients, B.1.3.1, Table B.1-3; results in the elderly, B.4.2.1, Table B.4-1; results in women, B.3.2.1

scavenger cell pathway, E.1.2, E.2.2

screening for dyslipidemia: in adults, ILIB, 2.1; in adults, NCEP, Table A.1-1; in children and adolescents, B.2.2, B.2.3, Table B.2-1; in diabetic adults, B.1.4

secondary dyslipidemia: causes of, 2.5; in children, B.2.3

secondary prevention of CHD: case studies, 3.9, 3.10, 3.12; clinical definition, 2.1; exercise, Tables D.4-1–D.4-3; transdermal nicotine in, Table D.5-1

SENDCAP (St. Mary's, Ealing, Northwick Park Diabetes Cardiovascular Disease Prevention) study, B.1.3.1

Seven Countries Study: plasma cholesterol and risk for CHD, 1.3.1; Mediterranean diet, D.2.2.3

SHEP (Systolic Hypertension in the Elderly Program), B.4.2

simvastatin: dosage, Table B.6-1; major lipid effects, Table B.6-2; use in FH, Table D.7-1. *See also* IDEAL; Scandinavian Simvastatin Survival Study

smoking: as major risk factor, Table 2.4-1; prevention in children and adolescents, B.2.2; risk in women, B.3.2

smoking cessation, Table D.5-1; antithrombogenic effect, Table E.2-1; case study, 3.2; in diabetic patients, Table B.1-2; lipid effects, Table D.1-1

sodium: maximum intake, Table 2.8-1

soy protein, D.2.2.7

SR-BI (class B, type I scavenger receptor), E.1.2, Figure E.1-2

SREBPs (sterol regulatory element–binding proteins), E.1.1

stabilization, lesion, 1.5.2, 1.6, E.2.4, Table E.2-2

STARS (St. Thomas' Atherosclerosis Regression Study), Table 1.6-1

statins. *See* HMG-CoA reductase inhibitors

Stockholm Ischemic Heart Disease Secondary Prevention Study, 1.5.2; results in the elderly, B.4.2.1

stroke: and estrogen replacement, B.3.4; prediction by PROCAM risk calculator, Figure F.1.1; prevention of first, Table F.1-2; reduction in risk for, with statin therapy, 1.5.2; risk factors for first ischemic, Table F.1-1

sulfonylureas, B.1.2, B.1.4.1, Table B.1-2

syndrome X, metabolic. *See* cardiovascular metabolic syndrome

thallium-201 imaging, exercise, 3.11

thiazolidinediones, E.1.3, Table B.1-2

thrombogenic risk factors, 2.4, Table E.2-1

tibolone, B.3.4

ticlopidine, Table E.2-1

TNT (Treating to New Targets) trial 1.5.2, Figure 1.5-2

trans fatty acids, Tables 2.8-1, A.1-7

transplantation, heart: use of statins with, Table D.6-1

triad, lipid, 1.3.5, 1.5.1, 3.3, 3.9

triggering of clinical events, E.2-4, Table E.2-2

triglyceride: delivery to peripheral tissues, E.1.1

triglyceride, fasting plasma: as CHD risk predictor, 1.3.3; risk in women, B.3.2. *See also* cutpoints, lipid; hypertriglyceridemia

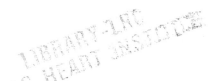

troglitazone, Table B.1-2

type I hyperlipidemia. *See* chylomicronemia

type III hyperlipidemia, 2.2.2, Tables 2.2-2, 2.6-1, A.1-5; and Friedewald formula, Table C.1-2

UCSF-SCOR (University of California, San Francisco, Arteriosclerosis Specialized Center of Research) Intervention Trial, 3.11; results in women, B.3.2.1

UKPDS (United Kingdom Prospective Diabetes Study), B.1.2

ultra⌐

unc

VA⌐

VL   ⌐.1-1,
E.1

wa⌐

wa⌐

wei   loes-
cer   3.4.4;
and   s for,
Tab

wo⌐   l dia-
bet⌐

Wo⌐

WO   derly,
B.4⌐

xan⌐

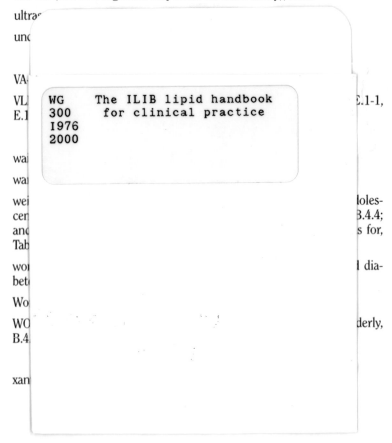